HORMONES

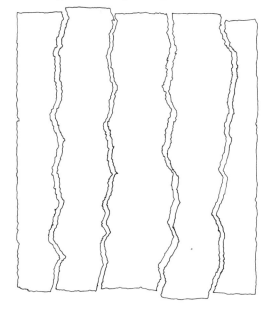

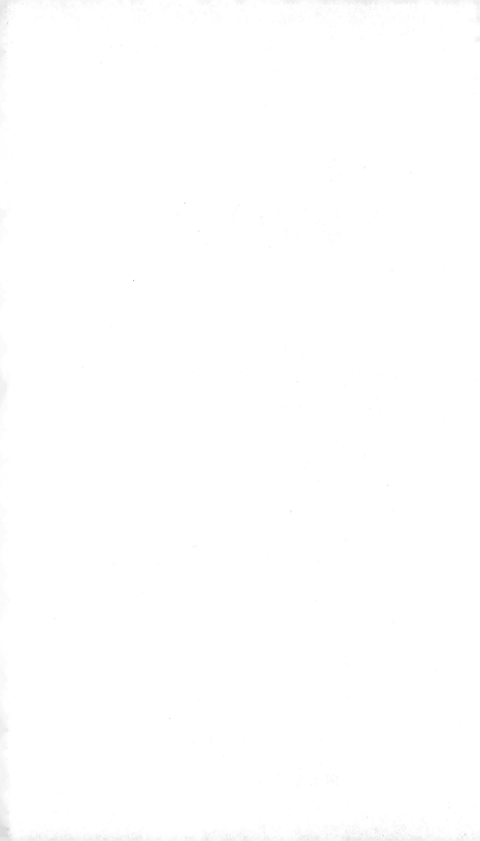

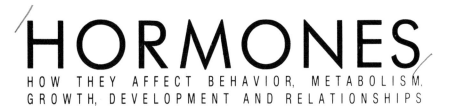

HORMONES

HOW THEY AFFECT BEHAVIOR, METABOLISM, GROWTH, DEVELOPMENT AND RELATIONSHIPS

by
Dr. Brian L.G. Morgan and Roberta Morgan

THE BODY PRESS
a division of
PRICE STERN SLOAN
Los Angeles

Notice: The information in this book is true and complete to the best of our knowledge. The book is intended only as a guide. It is not intended as a replacement for sound medical advice from a doctor. Only a doctor can include the variables of an individual's age, sex and past medical history needed for wise medical advice. Final decision about any medical action must be made by the individual and his or her doctor. All recommendations herein are made without guarantees on the part of the author or the publisher. The author and publisher disclaim all liability in connection with the use of this information.

Published by The Body Press
A Division of Price Stern Sloan
360 North La Cienega Boulevard
Los Angeles, CA 90048
© 1989 Price Stern Sloan, Inc.

Library of Congress Cataloging-in-Publication Data

Morgan, Brian L.G.
    Hormones: how they affect behavior, metabolism, growth, development and relationships / by Brian L.G. Morgan and Roberta Morgan.
        p.   cm.
    Bibliography: p.
    ISBN 0-89586-662-5
    1. Endocrinology—Popular works. 2. Hormones—Physiological effect. 3. Endocrine glands—Diseases—Popular works. I. Morgan, Roberta, 1953-   . II. Title.
QP187.M639 1989   88-39465
612'.4—dc19   CIP

10 9 8 7 6 5 4 3 2 1

CONTENTS

To our much loved and supportive families.

PART ONE

THE HORMONAL SYSTEM

CHAPTER ONE

THE BODY'S ORCHESTRA

Lisa was having a bad winter. The cold seemed colder than ever before and even several layers of clothing under her heavy sheepskin coat failed to keep her warm. She would close all the windows, turn the thermostat up as far as it would go, and wear bulky sweaters whenever she sat around the house. Her husband and children kept complaining about how hot it was indoors, but Lisa never seemed to feel warm enough.

It wasn't just the cold that was getting to her. She seemed to have almost no energy all of a sudden; cleaning the house exhausted her to the point where she had to take a three-hour nap in the middle of the day. She felt vaguely depressed much of the time, though she couldn't put her finger on what was wrong. And her skin seemed so dry and brittle it just soaked up moisturizers faster than she could apply them.

Her hair also felt unusually dry and started to look more like a fright wig than her normally shining brown locks. Then it began to fall out slowly. Later it became so noticeable that even her husband asked her if it was getting thinner. Lisa became frightened. Something was obviously wrong, but what was it? Her symptoms seemed vague and mild, and a few of her friends told her to forget about it and wait for the spring. "A lot of people get depressed and overly concerned about their health in the winter," her sister told her. "It's probably nothing to worry about."

It was the weight gain that finally drove Lisa to take action. After speaking with her friends and family and deciding her problems were all in her mind, Lisa vowed to take charge of her life, to see if she couldn't resolve her troubling symptoms through diet and exercise. She joined the local indoor pool even though swimming two laps suddenly felt like hiking thirty miles up hill. She even went on a strict diet. Lisa had always been proud of her figure and knew that if she just lost those few extra pounds she'd start to perk up again. But it didn't happen that way. To Lisa's amazement and then alarm, she began to gain weight! By the time the winter was almost over, she had put on fifteen pounds, even though she was eating less than ever before.

Her husband started teasing her about her "chubbiness." One morning, while sharing the bathroom, he looked over at her, grinned, and said, "You know, Lissy, even your neck is getting heavier." She looked more closely in the mirror and then drew back with a gasp. He was right. Her neck looked positively fat.

Lisa was at her wit's end. She went to see her family doctor, hoping he wouldn't think she was another middle-aged hypochondriac. He didn't. Instead, he sent her to a specialist who took blood tests and found that Lisa had a hormonal problem. Her thyroid gland was not working properly, causing the thyroid hormones in her body to be at seriously low levels. After several months on medication designed to correct those levels, Lisa completely recovered. Her hair came back, her weight returned to normal, the swelling of her neck went away, and the fatigue and depression disappeared.

Lisa hadn't thought she was sick, but it turned out she was wrong. Her body was out of balance, and that particular kind of imbalance, a hormonal one, can certainly be called a disease state. Some hormonal imbalances are actually serious illnesses. Lisa was one of the many people who've made a critical discovery: hormonal problems can cause very powerful changes in a person's body and mind.

WHAT ARE HORMONES?

Hormones can be thought of as chemical messengers that affect every cell in your body. They literally orchestrate almost all aspects of your life, from growth and development to metabolism and moods. They control such life-sustaining activities as your heart rate, respiration, digestion, immune responses, and your ability to respond to stress. Tiny quantities of these powerful substances are all that are required to keep the body in balance. Too much or too little can cause havoc. As we have just seen in Lisa's case, a drop in the body's level of thyroid hormone can cause your hair to fall out, your weight to increase, and your energy level to sink, making you feel fat and lethargic. Or, for another example, excess secretion of the hormone called cortisol over extended periods of time can lead to high blood pressure, heart attacks, and even possibly Alzheimer's disease.

WHY DO YOU NEED TO KNOW ABOUT HORMONES?

Many people like Lisa suffer from hormonal imbalances and don't realize they have a problem. Sometimes only vague symptoms will accompany a hormonal problem, even if the problem itself is quite severe. If you've noticed only slight symptoms, you might be tempted to say, "Oh, it's nothing," and not go for treatment. It is important to be attuned to your body, to recognize the signs of a hormonal imbalance and, if you have identified a potential problem to seek advice from a doctor who specializes in the field.

Of course, there is another side to this story. People are fond of blaming their glands for their problems: "I can't lose weight because I have sluggish glands"; or "My glands never make me feel sexy anymore the way they did when I was younger." The glands they are referring to are called the endocrine glands, which produce many but not all of the hormones found in your body. And sometimes, these glands are responsible for distressing symptoms. But it is important to be able to recognize when being overweight is a result of hormonal imbalance and when it is a result of too much food and too little exercise.

This book will help you sort out the signs and symptoms of hormonal imbalances so that you can gain a more accurate understanding of your body and its changes. Doctors frequently have to tell their patients: "Aging is not a hormonal problem, there's no cure for growing old." With today's emphasis on youth and fitness, however, many people panic when faced with wrinkles or reduced energy, even though these are simply signs of getting older. On the other hand, changes of skin condition and reduced energy could be a sign of a hormonal problem. So see your doctor if you experience troubling symptoms. Also, you can learn how to keep your body in balance to ensure healthier and better looking skin and hair. Learning more about your body and how hormones affect your life can help you identify when something has gone wrong and what you can do about it.

WHY DO YOU NEED THIS BOOK?

Besides helping you to recognize signs and symptoms of imbalances, there are other aims and purposes of this book. For example:

- Perhaps you have noticed that you have very low energy at certain times of the day, or are prone to headaches at times. In this book, you will learn how hormones affect how you think and feel.
- Perhaps you have been diagnosed as having a particular hormonal problem.
- Perhaps your doctor has been rather rushed in his explanation of the problem if he has even bothered to explain it at all. This book contains a Guide section that will answer your questions about the body's major hormones, their functions, and abnormalities.
- Perhaps you have noticed that under stress conditions you have difficulty sleeping, or even digesting your food, or that PMS is taking a great toll on your work every month. Sections of this book can acquaint you with ways you can lessen the effects of these hormonal problems.
- Perhaps a loved one is about to begin treatment for a hormonal imbalance, and your lack of information about the treatment has led you to believe this will be a terrifying procedure. In the Guide section of this book, methods of treatments are described so that you can reassure yourself and your loved one through knowledge. For example, to treat an elevated androgen level in a female, your physician may merely prescribe birth control pills.
- Perhaps you simply want to learn more about how your body works. This book's two parts, eight chapters followed by a Guide, can be used together to increase your knowledge.

THE STUDY OF HORMONES

The Chinese were the first to realize the importance of hormones (although they were not conscious of it at the time) when they used mineral-rich seaweed in the medieval era to treat people who had swollen necks, or goiters, due to an iodine deficiency. After that, nothing is documented about these mysterious chemical messengers until 1775 when Percival Patt, a surgeon at St. Barts Hospital in London, operated on a young woman to repair a hernia and inadvertently removed her ovaries. To his amazement, her breasts wasted away and her periods ceased. Another physician of the time, John Davidge, realized the importance of Patt's serendipitous discovery and wrote: "Menstruation is attributable to a peculiar condition of the ovaries, serving as a source of excitement to the vessels of the womb."

In the early 1900s, the name hormone (which means "to stir up" in Greek) was given to estrogen (secreted by the ovaries) and to other such substances that are released by the various organs and tissues of the body in order to maintain it in a normal state, with all of its millions of processes working in perfect harmony with one another.

In 1970, the scientific community could name only 20 hormones. Today, we know of the existence of at least 200 and the number is rising every year. In fact, we now recognize that almost anything produced by one cell that can get to another cell by any means and change what that cell does is called a hormone.

As we learn more about hormones we learn how to manipulate them so that we can improve the quality of your life. We can now insert human genes into bacteria to make them produce large quantities of hormones which are given to people who do not make enough of their own, such as diabetics. Insulin is now produced in this way, whereas years ago it was extracted from the pancreas of pigs or cows, a less efficient and time-consuming process.

Hormone research is opening up exciting new avenues of medical opportunity. Investigators are now looking into the possibility of producing hormones called thymosins, responsible for stimulating the immune system, to help AIDS patients. Synthetic hormones that stimulate cells to produce hair color may one day be used to prevent graying. Since hormones are known to influence behavior, research is actively being done in this area. Violent behavior may be the product of high sex hormone levels that could be corrected. The fact that we may age simply because a part of the brain called the hypothalamus loses its ability to keep our hormones and hence our bodies in perfect balance could lead to the discovery of how to retard the aging process itself.

THE GLANDS

Remember those endocrine glands everyone blames for their problems? They include the hypothalamus, thyroid, parathyroid, pituitary, pancreas, pineal body, gonads (the ovaries in women and the testes in men), adrenals, and thymus. Figure 1 shows you where they are located in your body.

We call them endocrine glands because they secrete their hormones directly into the bloodstream. Exocrine glands, on the other hand, secrete their fluids via little ducts (like tubes), not through the blood, to the outside of the body or to the inside of body cavities. Good examples of exocrine glands are the salivary glands in your mouth and the sweat glands. In this book, we will be concerned with the endocrine glands only.

Apart from these glands, many other body tissues (such as the hypothalamus and other parts of the brain, the kidneys, the heart, and the digestive system) also secrete hormones. Since these affect the internal balance of the body along with the endocrine glands, we will be examining them in greater detail as well.

The study of hormones is called endocrinology, and the physicians that specialize in hormonal disorders are called endocrinologists. As with all medical specialties today, the amount of knowledge about this area has grown so much in recent years that there are now several subspecialties of endocrinology such as reproductive endocrinology (dealing with conception and infertility), pediatric endocrinology (dealing with growth disorders), and neuroendocrinology (a new science concerned with the effects of the approximately forty-five separate hormones found in the brain).

HOW DO HORMONES WORK?

The numerous hormones of the body work in concert with one another and with the nervous system. This is why one imbalance can lead to others. When some part of this vast hormonal network goes out of balance a message is sent to the brain, which then responds by regulating the endocrine system to bring everything back into balance.

Consider, for example, a marathon runner. As the runner proceeds through the miles, he loses a lot of body water through perspiration. This alters the concentration of his blood, which is the signal for an endocrine gland, the hypothalamus, to release a hormone to correct this imbalance.

An imbalance in the bloodstream may also affect the endocrine system directly. For example, when your blood glucose level drops below normal, such as between meals, glucagon, a hormone produced by the pancreas, is secreted to raise blood glucose levels.

The endocrine system is a very effective way of amplifying small

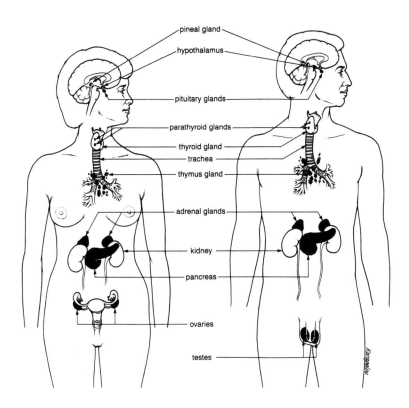

FIGURE 1 THE ENDOCRINE GLANDS

signals from the brain. For instance, the nervous system stimulates the hypothalamus (a small area set deep in the brain) to release small amounts of a regulating hormone into the blood system that joins it to the front of the pituitary. The pituitary then secretes a greater amount of hormones which are released into the bloodstream of the body. Each one of these hormones then specifically stimulates a different endocrine gland to produce even greater quantities of its hormones.

This chain of events is controlled by a very sensitive feedback system. Each part of the chain can cause increases or decreases in the hormonal secretions of another part simply by signaling it with its own hormones. Hence, the pituitary hormones can prevent the release of the hypothalamic hormones when their levels in the body become too high. This is called short-loop negative feedback. Long-loop negative feedback occurs when the hormones of the final targeted gland in the chain reduce the secretions of both the pituitary and the hypothalamus, again to prevent excessive hormonal levels. There is also positive feedback, where rising levels of a hormone cause even greater hormone release. For example, ovulation results from the effects of rising levels of estrogen causing the hypothalamus to produce greater amounts of gonadotropin-releasing hormone, which in turn stimulates the pituitary to release luteinizing hormone, which causes ovulation.

In the endocrine system, one hormonal messenger either wakes up or silences another, who then goes on to wake up or silence the next messenger, and so on, until the body reacts in a certain way. Thus, the hormonal system is itself kept in balance by the hormones it releases. They in turn keep the body's multitude of individual reactions operating at a suitable level to maintain our health and well-being. Any deviations from this perfect balance can lead to a progressive deterioration of the body.

This information is much easier to visualize when you examine one simple example of how it translates into everyday life. Let's look at the hormonal system of our marathon runner again. After the first few miles, he breaks into a light sweat. But after running half his course, perspiration has caused his body to lose quite a bit of water. His blood concentration goes up because his blood volume is going down. (When you lose a lot of water from the body, through perspiration to cool yourself off, this water has to be replaced by water from the bloodstream, therefore reducing blood volume.) When our marathoner's blood concentration goes up, his blood stimulates groups of cells in the hypothalamus called osmoreceptors. Once activated, these osmoreceptors stimulate the hypothalamus to produce a hormone called vasopressin. This hormone is passed down a group of nerves to the back of the runner's pituitary, which then secretes the vasopressin into his blood where it passes to his kidneys. The vasopressin makes the kidneys retain water, thereby protecting the runner from becoming dangerously dehydrated to the point where he cannot finish the race. The kidney's water retention causes the runner's blood volume to increase and its concentration to decrease.

But the runner's body does not use only one hormonal pathway to keep his blood volume and concentration normal. His reduced blood volume also activates cells in the wall of his heart called volume receptors. These pass messages to the hypothalamus via a nerve to notify it of the runner's reduced blood volume. In response, the hypothalamus produces even more vasopressin. This system is so sensitive that a change in blood concentration as small as 1-2 percent will cause significant changes in vasopressin secretion. Once the runner's blood volume and concentration are corrected, the stimulus for the production of vasopressin is removed and his hypothalamus stops releasing it.

Although this explanation is a somewhat simplified version of how the endocrine system works, it does illustrate the vital role hormones play in maintaining your body's normal balance.

HOW TO USE THIS BOOK

As far as this book is concerned, it is most important for you to thoroughly understand how hormones affect the way you think and feel. To ensure that this book has optimal usefulness as a resource, we have divided it into two distinct sections. In the first part of the book, The Hormone System, you will learn how hormones sustain life. We will discuss their role in regulating your appetite (and therefore your weight), in sex and sexuality, growth and development, behavior and moods. You will become acquainted with how hormones affect aspects of your life as varied as experiencing jet lag, having clear skin, and responding to stress. You will also discover how modern medicine is manipulating hormones to cure diseases.

The second section of this book is set up as an easy-to-use alphabetical reference, A Guide to Hormones and Hormone Problems. You can use this guide to obtain specific information on the endocrine glands, their hormones, their functions. The Guide explains what happens when the hormonal system goes awry, how you can know when something has gone wrong, and what can be done about it. Symptoms to look for in hormone diseases are described, as methods of treatment, what to expect when you see a doctor. We have included actual case histories, so that you can follow a patient's progress from diagnosis to treatment. The information contained in this book can be another tool in your work to keep your body in balance.

CHAPTER TWO

HOW HORMONES AFFECT THE BODY

Every body function is regulated to some extent by hormones. Even the functions of some of the hormones themselves are regulated by other hormones. It is a tightly integrated system. That is why when you are under stress from family problems at home and pressure at work, you not only experience anxiety but also notice disruptions in your sleep, your hair may seem dull and limp, high blood pressure, a stomach that seems to be under acid attack, and you may have recurring colds or flu. You may have other health problems too, of course, all influenced by hormones.

Hormones may either affect an organ directly, as in the case of the vasopressin in the marathon runner's bloodstream, or they may have no impact of their own but instead cause some other endocrine gland to go into action. This is exactly what happens with the trophic hormones produced by the hypothalamus; one of these is thyrotropin releasing hormone (TRH), which stimulates the pituitary to release thyroid stimulating hormone, which in turn stimulates the thyroid gland to produce thyroid hormones. Thus you can see that, in a system so interconnected, if one hormone is out of sync, others may be affected as well.

HOW DO HORMONES MOVE AROUND THE BODY?

There are two types of hormones, and they have different ways of moving through the body. Hormones are made from either protein or cholesterol (steroid). Those hormones produced by the hypothalamus, pituitary, gut, thyroid, and brain are all derived from proteins; those produced by the adrenal glands, gonads, the placenta, and the skin are all derived from cholesterol.

Protein-like hormones are stored as little granules in the cells within the endocrine glands that produce them. When they are needed by the body, they are pulled to the perimeter of the cell by strands of a muscle-like substance called actin and the hormone is expelled into the bloodstream. This phenomenon allows the gland to respond quickly to any demands for an increased secretion of hormones, because new hormone does not first have to be *made*, just taken out of storage. This is not the case for the steroid-derived hormones, however. The steroid hormones are not stored in cellular granules, so when more is needed additional cholesterol is picked up from the circulation, converted to the hormone, and then rapidly secreted into the blood.

Once in the bloodstream, any hormone moves with the blood until it encounters the specific receptor sites on cells that are programmed to recognize it and receive it. The protein-like hormones are too large to enter the cell itself, and so their receptor sites are special areas on the surface of their target cells. Once attached to the receptor site the protein-like hormone sets up a whole series of reactions that culminates in the production of a substance called cyclic AMP. This active molecule then initiates the series of actions regulated by that hormone.

A reaction of this type is very quick. For example, luteinizing hormone binding to the surface of cells in the testes makes them produce testosterone through the action of cyclic AMP, which activates the process. The end results are the secondary sex characteristics of the male (such as a beard, muscular build, and deep voice) and the production of sperm.

The steroid hormones are rapidly absorbed directly into their target cells and seek out a receptor site within the cell. The steroid hormone, bound to its receptor, then enters the cell's nucleus (which contains the genetic material of the cell) and activates the body's genes to carry out the hormonal action. For instance, your body needs calcium for healthy bones and teeth, along with other vital physical processes. At lunch time you might take in calcium through your diet, by eating a cheese sandwich and frozen yogurt (dairy products). But how does your body absorb this calcium from the food? It does it through the action of vitamin D, a steroid hormone made in your skin and activated in your liver and kidneys. Vitamin D stimulates the cells lining the walls of your intestine which are responsible for absorbing calcium to produce a carrier protein, which functions like a bus. This "bus" then moves the calcium from the food passing through your intestine across the wall of the intestine and into your blood stream.

Steroid hormones work more slowly than the protein-like ones because their action requires the production of new proteins by the cells. But what is the actual time difference between the two? Well, a process that would take two hours for a steroid hormone to complete would take only minutes for a protein-like hormone.

Now that we have some idea of how hormones work and how their levels in the bloodstream are carefully controlled, we should next look at our intricate endocrine system in greater detail. The remainder of this chapter is devoted to a brief view of the endocrine glands and some of the 200 hormones. Also, we'll mention only the major functions of each gland.

For a more detailed look at this system, see the tables in the guide section, pages 111—112.

THE HYPOTHALAMUS AND THE PITUITARY

FUNCTION (hypothalamus): The regulator glands; controls the pituitary.

FUNCTION (pituitary): The master gland; controls many of the other glands and processes.

HORMONES (hypothalamus): Trophic hormones; growth hormone releasing hormone (GnRH); many others. See Guide.

HORMONES (pituitary): Prolactin; growth hormone; vasopressin; many others. See Guide.

The hypothalamus lies in the brain under the front portion of your cerebral cortex (the thinking center), behind the nasal cavities. Although smaller than a fingertip and weighing just a quarter of an ounce it performs more tasks than any other brain structure of comparable size. It regulates body temperature; controls thirst and appetite; influences blood pressure, sexual behavior, memory, aggression, fear response, and sleep; helps to regulate our other emotions; and controls the pituitary gland.

The pituitary lies just below the hypothalamus. In adults it weighs about half a gram. It is often thought of as the master gland, the leader of the endocrine system because its hormones control so many of the other endocrine organs. The pituitary is divided into two parts: the foremost part, or anterior lobe, is made up of glandular tissue producing seven different hormones; and the back part, or posterior lobe, is mainly nerve tissue that stores two hormones called vasopressin and oxytocin which are made in the hypothalamus.

The anterior lobe is connected to the hypothalamus by a copious blood supply called the portal system because it carries hormones from the hypothalamus to the anterior lobe. The posterior lobe is connected to the hypothalamus by a network of nerves that carries hormones (vasopressin and oxytocin) from the hypothalamus down to the back of the pituitary.

To see how these methods of transport differ, let's compare them to the two ways a person might use to send a message to someone else. In the case of the posterior lobe, the message (the hormone) is sent from the person's home (the hypothalamus) directly, through the telephone lines (the nerve cells) to its recipient (the posterior pituitary). In the case of the anterior lobe, the message (the hormone) is dropped from the person's home (the hypothalamus) into the water (the portal system) where it floats downstream to its destination (the anterior pituitary).

Hormones must come in a releasing and an inhibiting form. For example, if there were no inhibiting factor to prevent the continuous release of prolactin, a woman's breasts would constantly produce milk. The releasing hormone or "on" switch, in this case, is the hormone PRF or prolactin releasing factor and the inhibiting hormone, or "off" switch, is PIH, prolactin release inhibiting hormone. The hypothalamus determines the timing of the onset of puberty by secreting gonadotropin releasing hormone; it produces two other hormones, oxytocin and vasopressin, which are passed down to the posterior pituitary to be secreted as needed. Oxytocin maintains the contractions of the uterus after labor has started in the pregnant woman and stimulates the breast to eject milk during breastfeeding. Vasopressin helps maintain the concentration and volume of the blood by its action upon the kidneys.

The hypothalamus also produces endorphins, enkephalins, and dynorphins which have various functions in the control of stress, appetite regulation, and pain thresholds. While endorphins are widely regarded as the body's natural morphine, controversy rages over their other functions. Some theorists believe endorphins control appetite and that there are specific endorphins for sugar intake and specific endorphins for fat, and so forth. Others disagree. Some theorists believe endorphins produce the "runner's high," whereas others think they determine a high or low pain threshold. Research has been inconclusive in these areas, largely due to the difficulty and expense of isolating endorphins for study.

Because the hypothalamus is connected to other parts of the brain as well as the pituitary, its control of the pituitary is greatly affected by physical and emotional stress.

Mark, an enterprising accountant, works late one night at his office and on his way home senses that someone is following him. As he speeds up his steps, the footsteps behind him also quicken. His brain now understands the stressful and possibly dangerous situation he is in and so relays to his hypothalamus the order to secrete corticotropin releasing hormone (CRH) into the bloodstream. His hypothalamus and pituitary are directly connected by blood vessels and so this hormone quickly reaches the pituitary, where adrenocorticotropic hormone (ACTH) is secreted. ACTH is then passed into Mark's blood supply and within a few seconds ends up in the adrenal glands where it causes the release of their hormones, the corticosteroids. These adrenal hormones protect Mark's body against the stressful situation by invoking the fight or flight response: his blood pressure rises, more blood flows to his muscles, and his energy level is stimulated. Through the action of these hormones, Mark becomes totally alert, stronger, and quicker and better able to deal with his dangerous situation. He now has the energy to outrun his potential attacker and make it safely home.

This stress-induced reaction is fine if you are running from an attacker, but not so fine if the stress is long-term and coming from your job or personal life. The body doesn't know the difference and so still invokes the fight or flight response. Over time, this raises blood pressure and blood fat levels dangerously, making you more prone to having a heart attack or stroke; impairing your immune system, making you more susceptible to infection; accelerating your rate of hair loss; and weakening your muscles and bones.

Obviously, the hypothalamus and the pituitary have far-reaching effects on many body systems. For example, too much growth hormone results in a great looking basketball player and too little causes the appearance of a dwarf. Too little gonadotropin-releasing hormone results in infertility. Too little vasopressin causes an insatiable thirst and over-production of urine. Fortunately, many of these and other hormonal problems can now be cured with hormone replacement therapy.

THE THYROID

FUNCTION: Affects growth; controls energy and mineral metabolism.

HORMONES: Triiodothyronine (T3); thyroxine (T4); calcitonin.

The thyroid gland, blamed for weight gain and loss among other sins, is fifteen to twenty-five grams in weight and shaped like a butterfly. It lies over the windpipe just below the larynx. The thyroid's hormones are essential to the activity of almost all the tissues of the body, and any deficiency or excess can have serious repercussions.

The thyroid hormones known as T3 and T4 speed up the activity of all the tissues in the body except for the brain, testes, anterior pituitary, and spleen. (The spleen is an essential component of the body's immune system; it is an organ that can produce red blood cells when the bone marrow is damaged and unable to carry out that function.) These hormones also speed up the body's ability to absorb and break down glucose and fat, which means that they lower cholesterol levels and reduce the risk of heart attacks. In addition, they have an essential role to play in the growth and development of children.

Thyroid stimulating hormone (TSH) from the pituitary stimulates the thyroid gland to make and release T3 and T4. A rise in the levels of T3/T4 hormones circulating in the blood exerts a negative feedback on TSH (thyroid stimulating hormone) secretion, whereas low circulating levels of T3/T4 result in a rise in TSH secretion. In other words, if the T3/T4 levels are too low, the TSH level will be high, and vice versa. This is how the amounts of thyroid hormones are maintained at a constant level in the body.

The other hormone released by the thyroid, calcitonin, reduces high blood calcium levels, which could occur after you have had a glass of milk or eaten some other food rich in calcium, by causing the calcium to be deposited in the bones and by increasing the amount lost in the urine through its effect on the kidneys. It is critically important to keep blood calcium levels constant in order to build and maintain the bones, as well as to keep the muscles contracting, the nerves passing messages around the body, and the blood clotting. Calcium is also needed to aid in many energy reactions. However, if a person has an excessive level of calcium in his body for an extended period of time he could get calcium deposits in the soft tissues of his body such as the arteries.

THE PARATHYROID

FUNCTION: Produces PTH to restore low blood calcium levels.

HORMONE: Parathyroid hormone (PTH).

Most people have four parathyroid glands, two on each side of the thyroid gland, one high and one low (close to the windpipe). All four are reddish-brown spindles about five millimeters long but varying in shape and size from person to person. Their only function is to secrete parathyroid hormone (PTH), which regulates the blood calcium level. A low level of blood calcium stimulates PTH secretion and the PTH then increases the body's calcium levels by its direct actions on the bone (causing bone to partially dissolve), the kidneys (causing them to excrete the phosphorus normally bound to calcium in the blood, so leaving them calcium free), and indirectly by enhancing the absorption of calcium in the intestines. If you don't have a high enough level of calcium in your body for a long period of time, symptoms such as muscular rigidity and excessive bleeding could appear. PTH secretion is, of course, inhibited by a rise in blood calcium levels.

THE THYMUS

FUNCTION: The ultimate controller of the immune system.

HORMONES: Thymosin.

The thymus lies behind the breastbone and is one of the several spots in the body where lymphocytes are produced. These cells form an important part of the immune system. The gland also produces a series of compounds known as thymosins, which appear to activate lymphocytes, making them capable of killing disease-causing microorganisms. The actions of thymosin are not completely understood at this time, but too much or too little of it in the body is believed to cause disease or to enable disease to be contracted.

Babies normally have a large thymus gland which continues to grow until right before puberty and then slowly shrinks until it becomes a fairly small gland in older adults. Babies born without a thymus are highly prone to infections but if they are given thymosin, the lymphocytes produced outside the gland (in places such as the spleen and bone marrow) become activated and the body gains normal immunity. Thymosin has also been given to elderly people who respond poorly to flu vaccine.

Let's imagine you have been suffering from long-term stress because of an employer whose inability to plan ahead to meet deadlines is exceeded only by his bad temper. You have had an earache for three weeks. Before that it was a hangnail that would not heal. What's going on? Why are you so prone to infection? It is partly because of the thymus. For some reason, during such adverse situations, the thymus shrinks and so produces less thymosin, reducing its ability to activate the lymphocytes capable of killing microorganisms.

THE GONADS

FUNCTION: Reproduction and sexual characteristics.

HORMONES: In women: estrogen, progesterone, and relaxin; in men: testosterone and related androgens.

At puberty, hormones secreted by the hypothalamus and the pituitary lead to the stimulation of the sex organs (the ovaries in women and the testes in men) which cause them to produce the sex hormones, responsible for the major differences we all know and love between men and women.

Gonadotropin releasing hormone (GnRH) from the hypothalamus signals the pituitary to produce luteinizing hormone (LH) and follicle stimulating hormone (FSH). In the female, these hormones stimulate the ovaries to produce estrogen, progesterone, and relaxin. In the male, they stimulate the testes to produce androgens (testosterone and other male sex hormones) and sperm.

The androgens are secreted at a steady rate and are responsible for the characteristics of masculinity such as the growth of facial hair, deepening of the voice, and increasing muscular development. They also affect the brain, making men on the whole more boisterous and aggressive. (Too much testosterone is believed to be a major factor in causing men to commit violent crimes.) Androgens are also produced in both sexes by the adrenal glands and control our sexual desires.

Estrogen and progesterone are produced in a cyclical fashion in women, and therefore they control the coming and going of the monthly menstrual period as well as the times of increased and decreased fertility. They make a woman's skin soft, help explain mood swings characteristic of premenstrual syndrome (PMS), give a woman breasts and shapely hips, protect her from heart disease until after menopause (a protection men don't have), prepare her body for pregnancy, and facilitate birth. Relaxin aids in the birth process.

THE ADRENALS

FUNCTION: Affect the fight or flight response; essential for metabolism.

HORMONES: Epinephrine; dopamine; cortisol; others. See Guide.

The two adrenal glands are each four to six grams in weight and sit like a three-cornered hat on top of the kidneys, the left one being longer and thinner than the right. Each gland can be divided into two parts: the medulla or inner part which produces catecholamines (epinephrine, norepinephrine, and dopamine); and the cortex or outer part which secretes the glucocorticoids (notably cortisol), the mineralocorticoids (notably aldosterone), and sex hormones (estrogen and androgens).

All actions involved in the fight or flight response mentioned earlier, as well as low blood sugar, exposure to the cold, low blood pressure, and exposure to altitude also stimulate catecholamine release by the adrenals. However, since catecholamines are produced by other tissues of the body a person can get by without an adrenal medulla. This is not true of the hormones secreted by the adrenal cortex, which are essential to normal body function.

Cortisol production is under the control of corticotropin releasing hormone (CRH) from the hypothalamus and ACTH from the pituitary. It is produced in spurts all the time but its levels are highest in the morning and lowest at night. This then explains our sleeping and waking patterns, but it has other effects as well.

Geraldine works for an advertising firm with offices on both coasts, and frequently finds herself flying cross-country. Though she has no difficulty sleeping on the plane, Geri is plagued by "jet lag" whenever she flies across several time zones. Researchers have found that it takes different amounts of time for our circadian rhythms (that is daily fluctuations of cortisol levels) to correct themselves. For most of us, it is a day for every time zone we cross.

Our circadian rhythm is mediated by CRH and ACTH which represent our biological clock. Furthermore, cortisol itself exerts a negative feedback on CRH secretion. Stress (psychological or physical) has the opposite effect and increases cortisol levels by increasing CRH secretion.

The sex hormones (estrogen and androgens) produced by the adrenals supplement those secreted by the ovaries and testes. Androgens produced in women also stimulate the growth of pubic and other body hair and increase a woman's sex drive. Adrenal estrogen is produced in only tiny quantities and has no known physiological significance, but it may prove to be important in certain diseases characterized by the appearance of feminine physical traits in the male.

THE PANCREAS

FUNCTION: Regulates the blood glucose levels.

HORMONES: Insulin; glucagon; somatostatin; and pancreatic polypeptide.

The pancreas weighs about fifty to seventy grams and lies behind the stomach with its head and tapering tail stretching across the vertebral column towards the left side, ending over the spleen. The pancreas is mainly concerned with the exocrine function of producing digestive enzymes which travel through ducts to empty into the intestine where they break down food.

The endocrine portion is only 2 to 3 percent of the gland and consists of two million cell structures called islets of Langerhans. These are groups of four different kinds of cells—A, B, D, and PP—which produce the hormones glucagon, insulin, somatostatin, and pancreatic polypeptide respectively.

Insulin is produced by the beta (B) cells which make up 80 percent of the islet of Langerhans. It is needed by almost all cells in the body because it enables them to absorb glucose, their main source of energy. Without glucose, the cells would die. When blood glucose levels rise after a person eats something sugary, the pancreas is directly stimulated to release insulin and the body is stimulated to produce proteins and fats.

Glucagon is secreted by the alpha (A) cells and stimulates the liver to break down its stored sugar (glycogen), which it releases into the body for use by other cells. When blood sugar levels fall, such as between meals, glucagon levels rise to ensure a constant supply of glucose to the tissues. Without this hormone, we would become comatose when the brain ran out of its main energy source. Glucagon also stimulates the production of glucose from protein.

Problems arising from a disturbance of the pancreatic hormones are among the most well known and at the same time most dangerous of endocrine disorders. The one we are all well acquainted with is called diabetes, and will be discussed in greater detail in chapter 3 and in the Guide.

THE PINEAL GLAND

FUNCTION: Produces melatonin, responsible for hair and skin color.

HORMONE: Melatonin.

The pineal gland weighs only one to two hundred milligrams and is situated right in the middle of the brain. It produces melatonin, a hormone that determines hair and skin color, and releases it primarily at night. The pineal gland seems to inhibit the secretion of gonadotropins and possibly other pituitary hormones but its complete role in the body remains undetermined at this time. One intriguing possibility is that it initiates puberty.

THE GASTROINTESTINAL SYSTEM

FUNCTION: Controls the secretion of digestive juices and the appetite.

HORMONES: Gastrin, cholecystokinin; secretin; others. See Guide.

The whole length of the digestive system contains a number of hormone-secreting cells and is perhaps the largest endocrine gland. (We have already mentioned the hormones secreted by the pancreas.) When we eat a meal, all of these hormones are released in a coordinated fashion as the food passes down the intestine. Either too much or too little of these hormones can cause serious problems, such as the inability to digest food as is the case when acid is not produced in the stomach (a condition known as achlorhydria, which can result in anemia due to the nonabsorption of iron). Ulcers can be caused when too much acid is produced.

THE KIDNEYS

FUNCTION: Help control blood pressure and blood manufacture.

HORMONES: Renin; REF.

The kidneys are instrumental in producing two very important hormones called renin and renal erythropoietic factor (REF). Renin is important for maintaining normal blood pressure and REF helps to control the production of red blood cells. When you go to a high altitude, or lose a lot of blood in an accident, REF causes your body to produce more red blood cells.

THE PROSTAGLANDINS

Unlike the hypothalamus or the adrenals, the prostaglandins are not endocrine glands but are hormones themselves. Though they cannot be neatly categorized, they are important to the endocrine system, and therefore are included here.

FUNCTION: Prostaglandins are involved in many if not all hormonal reactions in the body.

Prostaglandins are produced from a particular type of fat found in our diet called linoleic acid. The first time they were discovered was in the fluids produced by the prostate gland called semen (hence the term prostaglandins). Similar substances were later found in the kidneys, uterus, blood cells, joints, and many other tissues.

While prostaglandins appear to help carry out many hormonal reactions, they themselves are responsible for certain specific actions such as initiating labor, causing uterine contractions during menstruation, clumping together the blood cells called platelets during the clotting of the blood, and stimulating the immune system.

As with all the other hormones, a balance is required to maintain perfect health. An excessive level of prostaglandins may cause menstrual cramps or lead to strokes and heart attacks. Too little can result in high blood pressure and poor digestion.

CHAPTER THREE

RUNNING THE METABOLISM

Frank Davis, a man in his early 80's, phones his daughter and complains that every time he does any simple activity, such as working in his garden, he feels extremely tired. At first Frank's daughter shrugs it off as old age. After all, her father has been known to overdo it a bit in the garden. But then she notices cracks in the corners of her father's mouth and dark circles under his eyes. He complains that his tongue always feels sore. Frank's daughter becomes alarmed at her father's symptoms and brings him to the family doctor. After a blood workup, the doctor discovers Frank has iron deficiency anemia. The doctor explains that many older people suffer from this problem because they don't produce enough acid in their stomachs to aid in iron absorption. He prescribes intramuscular injections of iron.

What the doctor doesn't explain is that this is a problem of the metabolism and that Frank's anemia may be due to an inability on the part of the acid-secreting cells in his stomach to respond correctly to gastrin, a hormone produced in the stomach and upper part of the small intestine.

WHAT IS METABOLISM?

You have probably heard the word "metabolism" many times, but may have wondered what it means. Metabolism is simply everything that goes into keeping your body supplied with the energy it needs to stay alive and carry out its daily activities. Hormones have a very important role in supplying our bodies with this energy.

From the time food enters our mouths until it reaches individual cells, its passage is controlled and coordinated by hormones. And since our bodies obviously do not shut down between meals, hormones also supervise the extraction of those nutrients stored from the food we have eaten previously. This is also very important in situations where our body is called upon to do something outside our ordinary routine. For example, when we do some activity we are not accustomed to such as playing tennis for the first time in over a year we don't have to stock up on food just before the match because, again, hormones help the body draw on its stores of nutrients.

HOW HORMONES CONTROL THE METABOLISM

Hormones are responsible for keeping every tissue in the body supplied with the type of food source it specifically needs to fulfill its energy requirements. For example, the brain favors glucose while the liver can use glucose, fat, or protein. When your brain is deprived of its energy source, you may be unable to think clearly, feel weak and shaky (the brain also controls the muscles), and are more likely to make mistakes at work. You could also become anxious, easily upset, and depressed, your head may ache, and you may feel dizzy or nauseated. If you stop eating for two to three weeks, the brain can switch its energy source to a type of partially degraded fat called ketones (made in the liver) and start to function normally with a low level of glucose, but never without any glucose.

Many hormones are involved in the process of getting a continuous supply of glucose to the tissues (see Table 1), but insulin and to a lesser extent glucagon really control the energy supply. They are both present in the blood at all times and their levels are controlled by the level of blood glucose. When this level goes up, so does the level of insulin; when the level goes down, the amount of glucagon goes up.

TABLE 1
Hormones Involved in Getting Energy to Body Tissues

HORMONE	ACTION
Insulin	Decreases blood glucose, fatty acid, and amino acid level.
Gluagon, Epinephrine, Cortisol	Increase blood glucose and fatty acid levels.

HOW HORMONES REGULATE DIGESTION AND ABSORPTION

Before we discuss how specific foods are used by the body for energy, let's follow a meal down the digestive tract and see how hormones decide its fate. The food is swallowed and carried down the esophagus (the tube leading from the mouth to the stomach) by a muscular squeezing action that continues throughout the length of the digestive system. Once in the stomach, the food stimulates cells in its walls to secrete the hormone gastrin. This hormone passes into the bloodstream and stimulates other cells in the stomach to secrete hydrochloric acid.

Hydrochloric acid is so strong it can dissolve your tooth enamel. In fact, this is exactly what happens to bulimics, who repeatedly eat large quantities of food and then make themselves throw it up. The contents of their stomachs, combined with large amounts of acid, pass over their teeth and start to dissolve them. Our stomach lining is usually protected from the power of this acid because it is covered with a layer of mucous. However, when too much acid is produced, it can burn a hole in the stomach lining, which is what happens when you develop an ulcer.

The hydrochloric acid in the stomach has a big part to play in aiding protein digestion and a smaller role in the digestion of carbohydrates and fats. As more and more acid is produced, the stomach's acidity increases. When it reaches a certain level the gastrin-releasing cells are turned off, preventing the stomach from becoming too acidic.

The stomach then releases small amounts of food into the upper part of the small intestine (called the duodenum). Once this acidic, partially digested food (called chyme) comes into contact with the duodenal walls, another hormone, secretin, is released by cells within those walls.

Secretin passes into the bloodstream and circulates through the pancreas, stimulating it to release its digestive enzymes (amylase, lipases, and proteases) which digest sugars, fats, and proteins, respectively, and bicarbonate into the duodenum. The bicarbonate neutralizes the acidic chyme. Once this food is neutralized, the production of secretin stops. Without the continuous stimulation of secretin, the pancreas also stops releasing its digestive enzymes.

There is another step involved in this part of the digestive process. Any meal you eat contains some fat and when this fat enters the duodenum it stimulates the release of another hormone called cholecystokinin. This hormones travels through the blood to the gall bladder and stimulates it to squirt a green liquid called bile into the duodenum. The bile breaks the fat up into tiny droplets to form a suspension in the contents of the intestine, much like the oil in salad dressings. In this form, the fat can now be attacked on all sides by the digestive enzymes. Once it is broken up, the fat no longer stimulates the release of cholecystokinin and so the message to the gall bladder is canceled.

This two-step process means that fats take longer to digest than other types of food, and so the muscles in the intestine slow down to give them time. This delay is again under the control of the hormonal system. The fat stimulates the release of secretin and other digestive hormones (see Chapter 2) which suppress the nerves responsible for stimulating the muscle activity in the intestine that pushes food along its length. Everything slows down, and so the fat stays in the digestive system for several hours. Actually, its prolonged presence in the digestive system satisfies your hunger for a longer period of time, proving that some fat intake is useful when you go on a weight-reducing diet.

Once all the food is in the intestine, its walls secrete enzymes to help digest it. These enzymes, along with pancreatic enzymes, break down dietary carbohydrate into glucose, galactose, and fructose; fats into fatty acids and monoglycerides; and proteins into amino acids, all of which are absorbed into the body. Only fiber and other waste products (dead cells from the walls of the intestine, bile, water, and broken down enzymes and hormones) remain; they are pushed to the end of the intestine and passed out of the body as stools.

Your hormonally controlled digestive system doesn't develop fully at birth. An infant will spit out nonliquid food because of a protective instinct which tells her body she cannot yet digest solids. This is because her stomach's acid-producing cells do not respond correctly to gastrin,

TABLE 2
Simple and Complex Carbohydrate Foods

SIMPLE	FOOD SOURCE
Sucrose (contains glucose and fructose)	Table sugar Cakes Candies Molasses
Glucose	Corn syrup Honey
Fructose	Honey Dried fruit Fresh fruit
Lactose (contains glucose and galactose)	Milk

COMPLEX	FOOD SOURCE
Starch	Beans Breads Carrots Cereals Peas Crackers Nuts Pasta Potatoes Sweet potatoes

and because her pancreas produces only a limited amount of digestive enzymes when stimulated by secretin. When the infant reaches four to six months of age, the system begins to function properly and can accept the introduction of solid foods.

WHEN YOU EAT A MEAL

A normal American meal contains both simple sugars and complex carbohydrates (see Table 2). Glucose, fructose, and galactose are quickly absorbed, and the other carbohydrates are broken down into these three sugars and then absorbed. The rising concentration of glucose in the blood causes the pancreas to secrete more and more insulin. The insulin binds to specific receptors in the liver, muscle, and fat tissue where it helps the body absorb glucose for one to two hours after the meal.

About 30 percent of the carbohydrate coming into your body from your diet is grabbed by the liver, where all sugars are converted to glucose. The other 70 percent is used by your other tissues, especially the brain and red blood cells, which need a continuous supply. Anything remaining is broken down mostly by muscle and a little is converted into fat tissue.

Through the influence of insulin, much of the glucose reaching the liver and muscles is made into glycogen and stored for later use. Glycogen is composed of long chains of glucose molecules connected together. It's like storing freshly baked cookies in one tin in the refrigerator so you can remove them one by one when you are hungry later.

Protein is another matter. The amount you eat is broken down in the stomach and intestines and absorbed in the form of its constituent molecules, the amino acids. These also stimulate insulin production from the pancreas which causes them to be taken up by the tissues, to be used in making new body proteins. All parts of the body are subject to wear and tear, and so new proteins are needed constantly. The lining of the intestines needs to be replaced every 3 days, and your red blood cells wear out every 120 days. In fact, your body makes ten ounces of new protein each and every day. This amount not only includes the protein needed for tissue replacement and repair, but also for the manufacture of hormones, enzymes, and neurotransmitters (the nervous system's chemical messengers). When glucose is in short supply, new protein can be used as an additional energy source.

Fats are absorbed in their broken down form as fatty acids and monoglycerides. They pass into the liver and fat tissues where they are recycled into body fat again through the influence of insulin. This fat becomes an enormous storehouse of available energy. Whether you like it or not, about one-fifth of your body is fat. If you weigh 150 pounds, you are carrying around 30 pounds of fat, equal to an energy store of about 122,000 calories. Fat also protects our organs from everyday knocks and bruises, and forms an insulating layer under the skin to protect us from the cold.

WHAT IS THE BEST BREAKFAST?

To gain an optimum level of energy to start your day then, which of these foods, carbohydrates, protein, fats, is best? When you wake up in the morning, your blood contains 80-120 mg of glucose per 100 ml of blood. This is called the fasting blood glucose level and it is normal. If you don't eat after you wake up, the glucose level will slowly fall. When it gets down to about 70 mg per 100 ml, the lower end of the normal range, you will become hungry. If the meal you then eat contains some carbohydrate your blood glucose level will soon rise again. This is why the best kind of breakfast is one that includes carbohydrates, such as toast or cereal.

HOW HORMONES KEEP YOUR BODY RUNNING AFTER AN OVERNIGHT FAST

All of the glucose produced in the body after an overnight fast comes from the liver. When the level of glucose reaching the A cells of the pancreas falls below normal, these cells secrete glucagon into the bloodstream. When it reaches the liver the glucagon causes the stored glycogen to be slowly broken down in order to restore and maintain normal glucose levels.

Seventy-five percent of the glucose needed by the body is supplied in this way. The other 25 percent comes from newly made glucose. The liver uses breakdown products of glucose, protein, and fat obtained from other tissues to make new glucose. This process is called gluconeogenesis and is also activated by the hormone glucagon. In addition, glucagon causes the muscle to spare glucose by using fat for energy. (Muscle glycogen is never broken down to supply any other tissues with energy.)

Although only one-quarter of the glucose produced by the liver comes from gluconeogenesis, after an overnight fast the contribution made by glycogen soon decreases considerably and gluconeogenesis becomes more and more important as the fast continues.

When dietary carbohydrate is limited, or if food is not eaten following a twelve-hour fast, increasing amounts of fat tissue are broken down to produce fatty acids. These are delivered to the liver where they are broken down further to yield energy. The longer you fast or severely limit what you eat, the more fat is used for energy and the more ketones (partially broken down fat) are produced. Ketones may cause headaches in someone on a low carbohydrate reducing diet and can have further, more serious effects if they reach high levels, as with some diabetics (see the Guide).

PROBLEMS OF THE METABOLISM

There are a number of different ways in which hormones can cause your body's metabolism to function improperly and some of these problems are more serious than others. A hormonal imbalance can prevent the body from being able to absorb a vital nutrient: for example, as we saw at the beginning of this chapter, an inability of the stomach to produce enough acid can make the body respond incorrectly to the hormone gastrin and therefore interfere with the absorption of iron in the body, causing iron deficiency anemia. Other metabolic problems include hypoglycemia and hyperglycemia. But perhaps the most serious metabolic disorder is diabetes mellitus.

THE FACTS BEHIND HYPOGLYCEMIA

Hypoglycemia is the name used for abnormally low blood glucose levels. If your blood glucose levels drop below 70 mg per 100 ml and you still do not eat, the level will continue to fall as the glycogen stores in the liver are used up. Then you will experience all the symptoms associated with hypoglycemia—weakness, mental confusion and dizziness, and perhaps an intense craving for something sweet. If you give in to this feeling and gulp down a candy bar your blood glucose level will shoot up rapidly in response to the high sugar intake. Your pancreas will then secrete insulin to knock down the elevated glucose level. However, as many as one out of five women over the age of forty-five, along with a smaller proportion of people in the rest of the population, produce too much insulin and so the blood glucose level plummets, causing the symptoms of hypoglycemia to reappear. This problem is called reactive hypoglycemia and causes people to feel unwell much of the time, because their blood glucose levels are constantly bouncing from one extreme to another.

In order to avoid this problem, you should always eat when you are hungry and never wait until you feel famished. Unless you have an illness such as diabetes or obesity, hunger is a foolproof way of knowing your body needs more fuel.

WHAT IS DIABETES?

Diabetes mellitus affects people all around the world. A person with this disorder is unable to produce enough insulin in their body to allow the tissues to absorb the amount of glucose that is needed for the body to function. Damage to tissue in diabetics can lead to other complications, such as heart disease, vision problems, infections. Moreover hypoglycemia, or the inability to absorb glucose, in a diabetic can lead to coma.

Depending on the type of diabetes a person has, as well as the severity of the disease and a number of other factors including whether or not the person is overweight, the disease is treated through diet, drug therapy or a combination of the two. Diabetics must pay particular attention to what they eat and when to avoid hypo- or hyperglycemia. Generally, diabetics try to eat a daily diet containing 50-60 percent complex carbohydrates (which are rather slowly absorbed by the body and therefore only gradually increase blood sugar), plus about 20-30 percent fat and only about 10-15 percent simple sugars (which raise blood sugar levels very quickly and are therefore more difficult for the diabetic to absorb).

We have devoted a major section of the Guide to this common disorder. Please see the guide for more information including the types of the disease, early warning signs, methods of treatment, and a more specific discussion of dietary measures.

YOUR METABOLISM DURING STRESS

When you are under a lot of stress your body adapts to make sure you have all the energy you need to handle the perceived emergency. Epinephrine and cortisol are quickly produced and they cause the liver to break down glycogen as well as causing increased gluconeogenesis. This all serves to raise blood glucose levels and supply the brain with extra fuel. These hormones also increase the break down of fat tissue in order to raise fatty acid levels and so provide additional energy for the muscles. Glucagon secretion by the pancreas increases and insulin production decreases, again raising glucose levels. If you are running away from a man-eating tiger all of this is appropriate, but if the problem instead is a dictatorial boss the raised blood fat levels will merely increase your risk of having a heart attack or stroke.

YOUR METABOLISM DURING EXERCISE

Strenuous physical exercise places a special kind of stress on the body which causes a rapid increase in your need for energy. While at rest, 90 percent of muscle fuel comes from fatty acids and ketones. During the initial stages of strenuous exercise, the glycogen within the muscle is broken down and used. As this glycogen is used up, glucose is extracted from the blood passing through the muscle. The drop in blood glucose levels then causes the pancreas to secrete less insulin and more glucagon. The levels of norepinephrine, epinephrine, and cortisol in the body increase. As with stress, these hormonal changes stimulate the liver to produce more glucose and break down liver glycogen. They also promote the breakdown of fat to supply the muscles with fatty acids. When exercise stops, glucose levels increase, leading to a reduction in hormonal secretion.

As a long-distance runner, Sarah is particularly aware of the importance of glycogen to her performance. She knows that it is readily available as an energy source because it is present in the muscle itself, whereas fatty acids must first be liberated from her fat tissue and then transported to the muscle. Therefore, Sarah takes particular care to eat a diet extremely high in carbohydrates twenty-four to forty-eight hours before each race. She eats such things as pasta, lentils, potatoes, whole wheat bread, peas. This type of eating is called carbohydrate loading, or carbo loading, and its net result for Sarah is to increase the amount of glycogen in her muscle, giving her a readily available source of energy as she runs mile after mile.

BALANCING YOUR METABOLISM

Along with remembering to eat when you are hungry rather than waiting for desperate feelings of being famished, you should also make sure you consume only balanced meals, containing protein and fat as well as complex carbohydrate. The fat slows down the digestion and absorption of the carbohydrate so that it slowly trickles into the bloodstream and does not flood in, causing quick and dramatic rises in blood glucose levels. Protein causes the pancreas to produce glucagon, which diminishes the effects of glucose. Protein can also be broken down to produce substances the liver can convert into glucose should its glycogen stores become depleted. Therefore, working with your hormones, and for your body, means eating balanced meals at regular intervals. As we've seen, exercise can also help to balance your metabolism; as you walk or swim or play tennis, your body alters which hormones are being secreted and how these hormones break down nutrients into the required energy. Light and strenuous exercise have different effects.

CHAPTER FOUR

REGULATING THE APPETITE

Jerry had fifty pounds to lose before he would fall into the range of "ideal weight for this height." It was a frustrating process; already he had been dieting for three weeks. It seemed to him that no matter what he did, the pounds refused to slip away. Just yesterday, in fact, he had gone all day without eating. By the time he got home from work he was practically faint; he was forced to consume a whole bottle of orange juice and two hamburger patties just to keep himself from feeling dizzy or headachy. He added a cup of yogurt because he heard it was good for him. This dieting was really impossible. It was making him sick. Maybe he wasn't a pudge after all. Maybe he had a hormone problem . . .

Annie was sick and tired of hearing people always giving her advice on how to "gain those needed pounds." Always there were suggestions about milkshakes or protein supplements or adding an extra meal. Before they were always on her case about losing weight, losing weight. Now they were always bothering her with you're too thin, you're too thin. What did they want from her anyway? What was the value of eating all those fats and risking heart disease? Besides, probably this didn't have anything to do with weight anyway. Probably this was a hormone problem . . .

It is not uncommon to hear overweight or underweight people say that they are the way they are because they have an endocrine problem. In fact, many such people see their doctors complaining of a hormonal imbalance only to find that they simply eat too much or too little or all the wrong foods. While a disruption in normal hormonal functioning certainly can result in either obesity, as with Cushing's syndrome or hypothyroidism (see the Guide) or excessive weight loss, as with hyperthyroidism (see the Guide), most people merely have to face the fact that they must better regulate their diet to stay at an ideal weight.

However, this is not to say that hormones have nothing to do with your appetite: quite the contrary, in fact. Hormones are working in your body every minute to decide what and how much you should eat. The hypothalamus literally controls your appetite, and it is influenced in this function by hormones produced in the gastrointestinal tract and the adrenal glands.

THE HYPOTHALAMUS AND ITS CONTROL OF HUNGER

Many years ago scientists found that rats who had suffered damage to an area known as the lateral hypothalamus ate less food and gained less weight than normal animals. By contrast, they found that rats with damage to a different area, the ventromedial hypothalamus, ate way too much and became extremely obese. The animals with lateral damage acted as though they had absolutely no interest in food whereas the ones with ventromedial damage just couldn't satisfy their appetites. This research led to the "dual center" theory of feeding behavior. How much food you eat was thought to be controlled by a feeding center located in the lateral hypothalamus and a satiety center located in the ventromedial hypothalamus.

Since the time of this early research, many substances have been shown to have an effect on appetite by influencing these two centers in the hypothalamus. For example, glucose and fatty acids have a direct effect on the hypothalamus. Glucose seems to impair the appetite while fatty acids increase it. Brain-made hormones called endorphins and amino acids (the building blocks of protein) act both directly on the hypothalamus as well as on the gland's content of serotonin and norepinephrine, the chemical messengers called neurotransmitters that cause us to feel satiety or hunger, respectively. Endorphins increase appetite, amino acids decrease it.

Several hormones released by the gastrointestinal tract as food

TABLE 3
Hormones Known to Control Appetite

HORMONE	AFFECT ON APPETITE	SITE OF PRODUCTION
Glucagon	Decrease	Digestive tract
Somatostatin	Decrease	Digestive tract
Bombesin	Decrease	Digestive tract
Insulin	Increase	Digestive tract
Calcitonin	Decrease	Thyroid gland
Thyrotropin releasing hormone	Decrease	Hypothalamus
Corticotropin releasing hormone	Decrease	Hypothalamus
Prostaglandins	Decrease	Throughout the body
Endorphins	Increase	Hypothalamus and pituitary
Enkephalins	Increase	Brain
Cholecystokinin	Decrease	Brain and digestive tract
Cortisol	Decrease	Adrenal glands

passes down its length also signal the brain to feel satiety. Cholecystokinin (CCK) is one of these. It is released from the upper part of the small intestine and has its greatest effects five to fifteen minutes after the beginning of a meal. Its release appears to be mainly stimulated by the presence of two amino acids, tryptophan and phenylalanine, in the duodenum. CCK doesn't change your initial reaction to food, but rather appears to speed up the point at which you become full. Studies have found that people who have been given CCK on an experimental basis stop eating sooner but feel fully satisfied.

Other hormones known to affect appetite are listed in Table 3.

In addition to hormones affecting the appetite on a meal-to-meal basis, the amount of glucose being used by the hypothalamus also has an effect. When blood glucose levels drop, the glucose available for use by these cells drops and you feel hungry. You may be able to ignore these pangs for a while but they will eventually become overpowering. If you force yourself to eat nothing for a day or two, you may end up overeating because of ravenous hunger, thereby taking in even more calories than you would by eating normally. Well-spaced meals ensure that your blood glucose levels never fall too far below normal and so produce intense hunger pangs. This is a good thing for dieters to keep in mind. The other type of eating, starving and then overeating, often causes problems in weight loss. Many people complain that they haven't eaten a thing all day, suffered from terrible pangs of hunger, and still gained weight. On closer examination you would find that the person ate only a few hundred calories during the day but became so ravenous at night he consumed 3000 or 4000 calories in one sitting!

WHAT ARE EATING DISORDERS?

There are three basic eating disorders, or ways of eating that produce something other than a normal weight and energy supply. The first is obesity. Thirty-four million Americans suffer from this problem, which is defined as the state of being 20 percent or more over your ideal weight, based on height, frame, and sex (see Table 4). (There are a few exceptions to the rule, for example, body builders and football players, who are 20 percent or more over ideal weight due to an enormous amount of muscle, are not obese.) Being overweight is more than just a cosmetic problem; it creates an enormous psychological burden, and being five percent or more over your normal weight increases your risk for getting cancer, heart attacks, diabetes, lung disorders, gout, and arthritis.

Conversely, there are people who eat too little to maintain their lowest desirable body weight. They suffer from a disorder known as anorexia nervosa, which afflicts one out of every two hundred American girls between the ages of twelve and eighteen, as well as some boys and older people. Any kind of stressful event seems to trigger the disease, such as academic pressures, the fear of puberty, peer and parental pressures, marriage, divorce, a new job, or the birth of a child. Most anorectics have been overweight at some time in their lives and initially lose weight to get back to the ideal. But this reduction in weight becomes an obsession, and the person lives in total fear of gaining any weight back at all. The dieting can go to such extremes that some anorectics weigh as little as seventy pounds. Some even die, if they don't get professional help in time.

Finally, there is bulimia, where the person goes on uncontrollable eating binges followed by self-induced purging (by vomiting or using laxatives). Obsessed with becoming thin and not gaining weight,

TABLE 4
Ideal Weight for Height

Men

Height		Small Frame	Medium Frame	Large Frame
Feet	Inches			
5	2	128-134	131-141	138-150
5	3	130-136	133-143	140-153
5	4	132-138	135-145	142-156
5	5	134-140	137-148	144-160
5	6	136-142	139-151	146-164
5	7	138-145	142-154	149-168
5	8	140-148	145-157	152-172
5	9	142-151	148-160	155-176
5	10	144-154	151-163	158-180
5	11	146-157	154-166	161-184
6	0	149-160	157-170	164-188
6	1	152-164	160-174	168-192
6	2	155-168	164-178	172-197
6	3	158-172	167-182	176-202
6	4	162-176	171-187	181-207

Women

Height		Small Frame	Medium Frame	Large Frame
Feet	Inches			
4	10	102-111	109-121	118-131
4	11	103-113	111-123	120-134
5	0	104-115	113-126	122-137
5	1	106-118	115-129	125-140
5	2	108-121	118-132	128-143
5	3	111-124	121-135	131-147
5	4	114-127	124-138	134-151
5	5	117-130	127-141	137-155
5	6	120-133	130-144	140-159
5	7	123-136	133-147	143-163
5	8	126-139	136-150	146-167
5	9	129-142	139-153	149-170
5	10	132-145	142-156	152-173
5	11	135-148	145-159	155-176
6	0	138-151	148-162	158-179

Note: The above figures give the weights of people who live the longest. (Used by permission of Metropolitan Life Insurance Company)

bulimics go on prolonged fasts, exercise excessively, and take diet pills to stop any possible weight gains from the binge eating. Most bulimics are single, college-educated women in their early to mid-twenties, but some are older, younger, and/or male. Emotional stress, depression, boredom, or loneliness can trigger this illness, and it also can end in death if left untreated.

HORMONES AND ANOREXIA NERVOSA

Cortisol, bombesin, and endorphins may be involved somehow in the development of anorexia nervosa. All three hormones have been found to be at abnormally high levels in people with this problem. Cortisol and bombesin both inhibit appetite and so it is logical that high levels can severely suppress the appetite in an anorectic. Endorphins are the body's natural morphine. It has been found that endorphin levels go down when people eat. It might just be that anorectics deprive themselves of food to maintain these levels at an inflated point because they are addicted to the "high" endorphins provide. Further research will either prove or disprove this theory.

HOW TO CONTROL YOUR APPETITE

The control of appetite and body weight is clearly a very complex issue. A large number of factors affect the functioning of the hypothalamus directly, and so influence our feelings of hunger or satiety. In addition, taste, smell, and other environmental factors such as food advertisements all have some impact on what and how much we eat. Clearly, the control of body weight is not just a matter of "willpower" or poor eating habits. It is largely the domain of the hypothalamus. But is there anything we can do?

SHORT-TERM APPETITE CONTROL

You have probably seen dieting "helpers" on the market, products that are supposed to control your appetite. But just what is the theory behind these products. Well, when the stomach is severely distended, as it can be when you eat a very large meal, the stretched walls send messages to the hypothalamus that signal satiety. However, this mechanism doesn't work unless the stomach is so full that you feel uncomfortable. Therefore, the appetite suppressants on the market are mainly indigestible fiber. When eaten, these products, containing pectin or guar gum, swell as they absorb water in the stomach and thereby stretch it. These same substances can cause feelings of satiety in the intestine in smaller amounts. Products containing cellulose, bran, or other types of fiber are much less effective, since they don't absorb very much water.

LONG-TERM APPETITE CONTROL

There are many theories offered to explain how the hypothalamus keeps us within our correct weight range. One is that the body attempts to maintain its muscle mass at a constant level. The level of amino acids in the blood is proportional to the muscle mass and so when this drops below a certain point, indicating a drop in muscle mass, a person's appetite increases to correct this situation.

Another theory states that the hypothalamus stimulates appetite just enough to maintain the level of body fat at a set point or constant level. Interestingly, if you give a nondomesticated animal all it wants to eat, it will take in just enough to maintain its body weight. If you force-feed such an animal it will get fatter, but the moment the force-feeding stops it will begin to eat less than normal until it reaches its set weight again. If the animal is semistarved it will lose weight, but as soon as it is again given free access to food, it will eat more than normal until it has gained back the weight it has lost and no more. This stable, normal weight is called the set point.

A similar situation occurs in humans. Consider the case of Suzanne:

When Suzanne was in college, she found that no matter how much she ate (within reason), her weight never went over 105 pounds nor under 95 pounds—her set point. When she was in her late twenties, she found herself stabilizing at about 108 pounds, and it was difficult to get down to 105 again. In her late thirties she weighed about 119 at most times, and while she could diet down to 110, 95 was out of the question unless she wanted to feel vaguely sick and fatigued all the time. What had happened was that Suzanne's set point changed with advancing age.

Fat cells are also involved in the appetite. Body fat is made up of millions of individual fat cells. Most are acquired during early childhood, pre-adolescence, and adolescence, but small increases can occur at any time in a person's life. Once you have these cells, you don't lose them. The cell size is elastic, however, and depends on how much fat is stored within it.

Fat cells are always releasing fatty acids into the bloodstream. These substances are absorbed by other tissues for energy purposes. During a fast, larger quantities of fatty acids are pumped into the blood. It has been hypothesized that as the level of fatty acids passing through the hypothalamus increases, the gland is triggered to increase the appetite. As your fat cells release fatty acids during the fast they become progressively smaller and you lose weight. When you eat normally again, extra calories are consumed and stored as fat in the fat cells. However, the cells continue to release higher than normal amounts of fatty acids until they return to their pre-fasting size, which means that your appetite is maintained at a higher level until the fat cells return to normal size and the body returns to its fixed point.

People who have a weight problem usually have larger and more fat cells than naturally lean people; in fact, their cells may be as much as two and a half times larger. If they reduce their fat cell size to normal by dieting they may still be overweight because they have so many more cells. The only way they can weigh the same as a lean person is to reduce their fat cell size below normal. As we just explained, when the fat cell size is decreased too much, the amount of fatty acids released is elevated, and the appetite increases. This is probably the reason why people who have to diet feel hungry most of the time when they are down to their ideal weight. These people also use the energy from their food very efficiently, as the body's energy conservation mechanism is turned on when fat cell size decreases below normal. Unfortunately, this means that these people need fewer calories than naturally lean people to maintain a normal weight (perhaps as much as 25 percent less).

Shelley, a twenty-five-year-old graduate student, had yet to be asked out on a date. She'd always been an attractive girl, with bright red hair and sparkling green eyes, always ready with a joke or a word of support for a friend. But she was also fifty pounds overweight. The other girls in her dormitory would drive her almost to tears when they would tell her to just eat less; eating less was exactly what she did. Shelley kept herself on a diet almost all the time and always felt hungry and tired. She noticed that she ate about half what her slim roommate did, but to no avail. Finally, on one of her many lonely weekend nights, Shelley decided to seek the help of a professional nutritionist. He explained why it was so difficult for her to lose weight: since she had been overweight right from childhood, she probably had many large fat cells. He also explained that this didn't mean she had to stay heavy. He put her on a well-balanced meal plan and started her on an exercise program. The slight modifications in diet, coupled with the all-important exercise regimen, brought Shelley down to a normal weight within a year.

FAT CRAVERS

In continuing to research the appetite, scientists have made a number of discoveries that may prove helpful one day. For example, people who are overweight show a definite preference for foods that are high in fat and carbohydrate content and have less of a liking for high protein foods. Scientists have shown in animal experiments that the craving for fatty foods is caused by brain endorphin levels. Obese animals were found to have higher levels of endorphins in their hypothalamus and larger appetites. When drugs like naloxone (which neutralizes the effects of endorphins) were given to them, their appetite decreased. Mild stress sometimes increases appetite in animals and when it does, it also raises brain endorphin levels.

TREATING AN EATING DISORDER

Though there are no instant solutions, we can help ourselves stay at an ideal weight by eating balanced meals, taking regular exercise, and recognizing when we do have a weight problem so we can adjust our eating habits to correct it. If you're overweight, this means eating smaller portions, reducing the number of snacks you consume, and increasing the amount of exercise you do in a week (at least one half-hour three times a week is recommended, but see your doctor first before beginning any type of strenuous exercise program). If you are dieting, you should always aim for a weight loss of no more and no less than one to two pounds a week. It is not wise to follow a crash diet, as such programs are usually not based on sound nutritional information and do not keep weight off permanently. They can also cause deficiencies in vital nutrients and lead to severe health problems.

There is no cure at this point for anorexia nervosa or bulimia. These patients usually need to be hospitalized, where they can be force-fed if necessary, given intensive psychotherapy, and sometimes treated with antidepressant medications. In the future, however, manipulation of elevated hormonal levels in these patients as well as obese patients may lead to different alternatives for treatment.

CHAPTER FIVE

EFFECTS ON GROWTH AND DEVELOPMENT

Both Roseanne and her husband were somewhat short. And though she sometimes enjoyed being considered petite, Roseanne also would become annoyed in clothing stores when the only outfits available were pink and doll-like or made her look "cute." She felt she could be sophisticated, too. Her husband Ed was a high school teacher; he occasionally felt as if the behavior problems he had with some of his students was that they didn't take him seriously because he wasn't as tall as they were. When their children were born, Roseanne and Ed pored over all the charts describing "normal" height and weight for infants at three months, at six months, at nine months. They weren't obsessed, but they sincerely hoped that their kids would fall into the upper percentiles. Yet in elementary school, it looked as if both children were going to be among the smaller ones in their age groups. When Roseanne and Ed confided to their pediatrician that they wished their children would grow more, they were surprised at the doctor's response. "Make sure they're not sneaking late night TV in their rooms at night," she said. "They need plenty of rest and the right diet. Enroll them in after school sports and exercise programs. Exercise stimulates growth hormone."

The growth of the human body is a very complicated process that is affected by hormones, as well as genetics, nutritional status, altitude, and various illnesses. In fact, the very term "growth" refers to different things. Your height depends on how much your skeleton grows, but your growth also refers to increases in the size and numbers of cells in all tissues throughout the body. In the end, however, the final size a person grows to depends largely on how quickly and how long he grows, both of which are under the control of hormones.

HOW THE BABY GROWS IN THE WOMB

By the tenth week of pregnancy, all of the body's organs are present in the unborn fetus despite the fact that it only weighs three grams (a tenth of an ounce) and is three centimeters (a little over an inch) in length. From this point onwards, it grows very rapidly, reaches its peak at twenty weeks, and then gradually slows down to a slower rate of growth until the end of the pregnancy.

Fetal growth is affected only to some extent by hormones, mainly insulin, thyroid hormone, and a hormone called placental lactogen. It is influenced more by genetics and other contributing factors. For example, infant size is very much affected by the size of the mother. Large mothers tend to give birth to large babies and small mothers to small babies. Male babies also tend to be larger than the females. Twins are smaller than babies born alone. Teenage mothers and mothers over the age of thirty-eight having their first child generally have smaller babies.

The differences that genetics can make in a baby's size may be most easily seen by comparing the average birthweight of different homogeneous populations. The average birthweight of Cheyenne Indian children is eight pounds, five ounces, whereas the children of the Luni tribe of New Guinea weigh on average about five pounds, four ounces at birth.

HOW THE BABY GROWS AFTER BIRTH

After the baby is born, hormones have a very important role to play in the growth process, as we will soon see. However, genetics and nutritional factors are also very important. If the baby is not fed enough it will not grow well. If the parents and grandparents are small, the child is unlikely to top six feet. For example, one of the authors of this book has a mother who stands 5'5" and a father who is 5'11". The author is 6'. The other author is a little over 5' tall; her mother is only 4'10" and her father is 5'5".

During the first year of life, children grow very rapidly; in fact, they increase their body length by 50 percent. Then, a year or two after this, the growth rate drops off sharply and stays lower until puberty, when it spurts up again. In fact, during childhood, growth occurs at a rate of two to three inches a year but during adolescence, height increases by 25 percent and body weight almost doubles. That is why your children seem to grow so quickly when they are first born, grow at a slower rate through young childhood, and really start to put on inches again during adolescence.

GROWTH DURING ADOLESCENCE AND BEYOND

During puberty, linear growth (height) speeds up again. It begins about two years earlier in the female (age eleven) than in the male (age thirteen). This means that boys, who also have a bigger adolescent growth spurt, have two more years to grow before entering puberty, and consequently tend to end up taller than girls. In both sexes the growth spurt lasts about two years, peaking at age twelve in girls and age fourteen in boys. These ages can vary, of course. Consider the case of Rory.

Rory hated high school from the very first day. He was so much shorter than the rest of his classmates he became the object of practical jokes. He couldn't play on the basketball team, girls avoided him, and the class bullies intimidated him at every turn. Seeing how unhappy he was and worrying that their son might take after his 5' mother and not his 6' father, Rory's parents brought him to the doctor. They asked the physician whether there was something wrong with their son and if anything could be done to make him grow.

The doctor took a growth history. At this point, Rory was fourteen years old, stood about 5'2", weighed only 111 pounds. At birth, Rory weighed a normal 7 pounds, 5 ounces. Throughout childhood, he grew at a normal rate, according to all the charts. By ten years old he was 4'6" and proceeded to add one or two inches to his height each year after that.

After some basic tests, the doctor brought the whole family in and explained that although Rory did seem short now, he was almost positive there was nothing to worry about. The boy was just about to embark on a growth spurt that takes place during puberty and the doctor was sure he would gain many inches during that time. As it turned out, the physician was right; by the time Rory graduated from high school at eighteen, he was over 6' tall and weighed 160 pounds. He played basketball in his freshman year in college and was a high scorer for his team.

At the end of puberty, the bones fully "mature," and growth in height stops for good. This happens at about age seventeen in girls and nineteen in boys. While you cannot grow any taller once your bones mature, hormones that affect growth are still operating in your body, where they influence your metabolism, as well as the growth of muscle and other body tissues.

THE MAIN HORMONES INVOLVED IN GROWTH

Several hormones, working alone and together, have an influence on growth. These include:

GROWTH HORMONE
The major influence on body growth after birth. It works by causing the liver and other tissues to produce hormones called somatomedins, that directly affect growth.

THYROID HORMONES
These have an important function in the development of the brain. They also increase the secretion and effectiveness of growth hormone.

ANDROGENS
In both sexes, the "male" hormones accelerate growth in height during adolescence, increase muscle growth, and accelerate the maturation of the bones and therefore the end of their growth.

ESTROGENS
In mainly women, the "female" hormones accelerate the growth and maturation of the bones.

INSULIN
This hormone stimulates the growth of the fetus, increases growth after birth, and increases the production of somatomedins.

CORTISOL
This hormone prevents growth.

GROWTH HORMONE

Following birth, growth hormone has the most influence on actual growth. One third of all the cells in the anterior pituitary are devoted to making this hormone. It is stored in sac-like structures (called vesicles) within the pituitary gland and is secreted when stimulated to do so. Throughout your life, two milligrams of this hormone are secreted each day.

Growth hormone has a number of jobs to do in the body. Before puberty, it stimulates the growth of the long bones in the arms and legs. Right on through adulthood, it stimulates the growth of the organs and other tissues and affects the metabolism. Between meals it helps break down fat to supply the body with energy. Growth hormone stimulates the production of protein in all tissues, for their maintenance and repair. In times of glucose shortage (such as during a fast), it increases the amount of glucose put out by the liver and decreases its use by the muscles so as to preserve any available amounts for the brain.

Growth hormone is thought to work by stimulating the liver and other tissues to make substances called somatomedins, which cause the actual growth. The production of growth hormone is ruled by the hypothalamus, which releases growth hormone releasing hormone (GHRH) and growth hormone inhibiting hormone (GHIH). GHRH causes the release of growth hormone from the anterior pituitary as well as stimulating the gland to make more growth hormone. When growth hormone and somatomedins reach a certain level in the body, they stop any more secretion by acting on the hypothalamus and pituitary. The hypothalamus produces GHIH which stops the release of growth hormone. Somatomedins also work directly on the pituitary, to prevent

GHRH from having any effect on the release of growth hormone. Thus you can see how, through using such a precise feedback system, the body regulates its hormonal levels.

There are other factors that influence the release of growth hormone. Factors that increase its secretion:
Sleep
Low blood sugar
Estrogen
Epinephrine

Factors that decrease its secretion
Obesity
High blood sugar
Cortisol

This is the reason why overweight children are often short and squat in appearance and why diabetic children may suffer from stunted growth.

The levels of growth hormone stay fairly constant throughout the day but one hour after falling asleep they increase a great deal, only to gradually fall again by morning. Babies sleep so much partly because they are growing. Adolescents sleep more during their growth spurt years. The ancient Chinese were the first ones to observe this correlation, noting that children who did not sleep well failed to grow properly.

Wendy, a thirty-year-old writer, barely reaches five feet in height, even though her parents are not abnormally short. However, throughout her childhood and early adolescence, she would sit up half the night making up stories and poems and rarely got more than three to four hours sleep. There is a strong chance that Wendy could have grown a little more if she had gotten more rest during those crucial years.

Exercise and all other types of physical activity stimulate the secretion of growth hormone, which is why it is a good idea to encourage your children to participate in school sports and exercise programs. Metabolic and nutritional factors also play a role. After a high protein meal, for example, growth hormone stimulates the tissues to make protein, resulting in an increase in muscle mass. Age also affects these levels: they are highest in the fetus even though the hormone is not needed for fetal growth; during early childhood the levels are similar to those of adults; they increase at puberty; go down after adolescence to normal adult levels; and gradually decline by old age.

GROWTH HORMONE DEFICIENCY IN CHILDHOOD

A deficiency of growth hormone in childhood can cut growth rates in half and result in dwarfism. However, since not all bone growth is equally affected, the head and face often become deformed. Growth hormone-deficient children also tend to be fat and have poorly developed muscles. Puberty is delayed. When adults have this problem, it causes reduced muscle strength, weak bones, and a tendency to low blood sugar.

There are 150,000 growth hormone-deficient children in the United States who receive growth hormone, which is made by adding growth hormone-producing genes to bacteria. The hormonal therapy works very well during the first year of treatment, but then rapidly becomes less effective.

Should growth hormone be used on short children who do not have a deficiency but whose parents want them to be taller? The answer is no, this is not a good idea. Even though growth hormone will speed up the growth of the bones it will also speed up the time at which they mature. As a result, the bones of these children may mature before they reach their genetic potential, and they can end up shorter than they would have been had they been given the chance to grow normally.

Too much growth hormone can also cause diabetes because it raises blood sugar levels. In rare cases, it has been known to make the thigh bone slip out of its socket in the hip, which can occur when the bones grow too quickly. The problem must then be corrected with major surgery. However, in the future, growth hormone may be used for adults in the treatment of wounds and fractures because of its ability to promote tissue growth.

INSULIN

As well as having a very important role to play throughout life in how the body handles glucose, insulin also promotes growth of the fetus. This may explain why diabetic mothers usually have large babies (weighing over nine pounds). Because the mother's body has high levels of blood glucose, the fetus' body produces large amounts of insulin to compensate. Not only is insulin very similar in structure to the soma-tomedins, and could conceivably mimic their growth-promoting actions, it also increases somatomedin production by the liver and other tissues.

THYROID HORMONES

Thyroid hormones are needed for normal brain development during the last part of pregnancy and the first two months after birth. Babies who are born to mothers with thyroid deficiency are usually of normal size but also thyroid deficient. If this is not found and treated very quickly, the child will develop irreversible mental retardation, because the brain will not grow properly.

Thyroid hormones are also needed for the growth of other tissues, including those of the skeleton. Unlike hypothyroid babies, hypothyroid children are very small because the actions of growth hormone are diminished. Thyroid hormones encourage the growth-promoting actions of growth hormones as well as increasing the secretion of growth hormone by the pituitary. Hypothyroid children have other symptoms of disturbed development, such as an abnormally large head, coarse features such as a pug nose and swollen eyelids, a short neck and thickened limbs. If thyroid hormone is given to the mother late in pregnancy and then given to the child after birth, these problems can be corrected. This is why pregnant women with any symptoms of thyroid disease (see the Guide) should see their doctors and take the appropriate tests.

A deficiency of thyroid hormone in later childhood will also prevent normal growth but here the child can catch up once he or she is given treatment.

ANDROGENS

Androgens produced by the adrenal glands in both sexes and by the testes in males are important to the adolescent growth spurt. They stimulate linear growth as well as weight gain and increase muscular development. (The latter effect explains why body builders and athletes sometimes unwisely take large amounts of these hormones, which can have such side effects as liver disease, high blood pressure, and sterility.) Androgens also stimulate the secretion of growth hormone by the pituitary and speed up the maturation of the bones.

ESTROGENS

Estrogen, at the normal levels found in the body, also speeds up the growth and maturation of bones. However, pharmacological doses decrease growth, possibly by reducing somatomedin production. Because of this, they are used to stop growth in very tall girls. Abnormally high levels of estrogen in girls (or androgens in boys) will lead to precocious puberty (see the Guide). These children will be very tall in their early years, but if the sex hormones are not suppressed and sexual maturation occurs, they will stop growing prematurely and end up being very short.

CORTISOL

Cortisol inhibits growth. This can be clearly seen in children with abnormally high blood cortisol levels (see Cushing's syndrome in the Guide) and in children treated with cortisol for asthma and arthritis. It inhibits linear growth as well as the growth of the muscles, liver, and kidneys.

SOMATOMEDINS

As we have seen, a number of hormones promote growth by raising the body's level of somatomedins. Age is another factor that affects these hormones: blood levels are low at birth, and despite a gradual increase throughout the first few years of life remain low until puberty. Somatomedins are not only made by the liver but by other tissues (such as the muscle and kidneys) as well, to promote their own growth, and this seems to be more important to development in the early years of life than does the amount of growth hormone circulating in the blood. At puberty somatomedins in the blood increase to two times the adult level, probably because they are crucial to the adolescent growth spurt. After puberty they drop to the normal adult level. The elderly have only half the amount found in younger adults.

Somatomedins are found in low levels in people with a growth hormone deficiency, and in high levels in people suffering from acromegaly or gigantism (see the Guide). They are elevated during pregnancy due to the action of a hormone called placental lactogen, which is produced, as you would expect, by the placenta. Certain illnesses, such as chronic liver and kidney disease, decrease somatomedin levels, which undoubtedly accounts for the fact that children with these disorders do not grow properly. Fasting also decreases soma-tomedin levels; there is not enough food to support the growth of new tissues. In fact, some anorectic children and adolescents do stunt their growth by not eating properly.

OTHER FACTORS AFFECTING GROWTH

A number of other factors affect growth; including:
- Fibroblast growth factor
  Affects the growth of cells throughout the body and is produced by the pituitary and other brain tissues;
- Epidermal growth factor (EGF)
  Produced by a number of tissues and also found in breast milk and the amniotic fluid (which surrounds the fetus in the uterus); some tumors produce EGF-like substances;
- Erythropoietin
  Produced by the kidneys, stimulates blood formation;
- Nerve growth factor (NGF)
  Important to the growth and development of the fetal brain;
- Thymosins, thymopoietins, and interleukins
  Stimulate the immune system.

PLATELET-DERIVED GROWTH FACTOR (PDGF)

Platelets (small blood cells) produce this substance, known as PDGF, which promotes another type of growth: the healing of wounds by causing the cells that form scar tissue to divide and increase in number. One theory states that PDGF is also involved in the develop-ment of atherosclerosis (hardening of the arteries). Damage to the walls of the blood vessels caused by deposits of cholesterol might attract platelets. These would then release PDGF, which would cause the cells in the wall of the damaged artery to grow, further blocking the passage and increasing the chances of having a heart attack. Recently, people who had suffered from a heart attack were advised to take one aspirin every day or every other day. This is because aspirin stops platelets from sticking together, which means that it stops PDGF from working in this destructive manner. Other scientists believe that PDGF may cause cells to grow inappropriately and cause cancer. Researchers are now trying to find ways to inhibit PDGF, and so possibly provide a form of treatment for these two leading causes of death in our society.

ALTITUDE

And finally, one other factor affecting growth has not yet been mentioned: altitude. It seems that people who live at high altitudes are not as tall as those who grow up nearer to sea level. This is because there is less and less oxygen the higher up you go.

IN CONCLUSION

As you can see, many hormones work together to bring about the growth and development of the human body. However, even if the hormones are all working properly and in balance, there are other factors that come into play in deciding how big a person will be, including food intake, genetics, birth location, and the absence or presence of certain diseases.

Perhaps the best way to predict the size of a child is to look at his or her parents and grandparents. There are two million children in the United States who are shorter than average, but the vast majority of them are normal and just genetically programmed to be small. However, the possibility of a hormonal imbalance should always be looked into if the child is either not growing as quickly as his peers, or if he is exceptionally small when his parents and/or siblings are not.

CHAPTER SIX

HORMONES AND SEX

Tall, trim, still athletic, with thick dark hair, John was one of those men who never seemed to age. You would never know he was sixty. He himself had never seemed to pay a lot of attention to growing older. He just naturally had always eaten well—low-salt, low-fat, high fiber diets fit easily into his life—and walking to work not only provided him with aerobic exercise, but gave him a chance to clear his head before having to face the demands of his customers, screaming their orders over the phone. But lately John felt as if he was losing his grip on his life. He didn't feel like leaving the house, much less having to trudge to work. Worse, he had to admit that his interest in sex was fading and almost gone. Maybe it was a serious disease, he thought. Maybe this was a sign of premature senility. "It's just the male menopause," John sighed. "Well then," said his wife, "it's all in your head."

Next door, Rebecca had just given birth to her first child, a beautiful girl, the child she and her husband had been waiting for, counting on. They had decorated the baby's room, bought books and toys to take the child all the way through the first grade, studied materials on child nutrition, planned future camping trips. The coming birth had filled them with such warmth, such excitement. But the day after the baby was born, Rebecca's usual high spirits completely vanished. She was

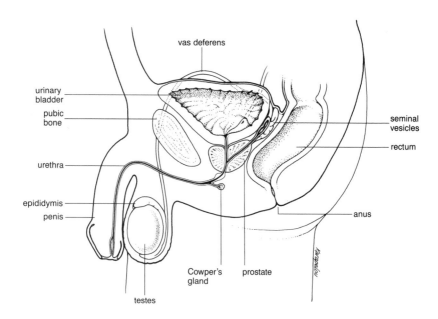

FIGURE 2 MALE SEX ORGANS

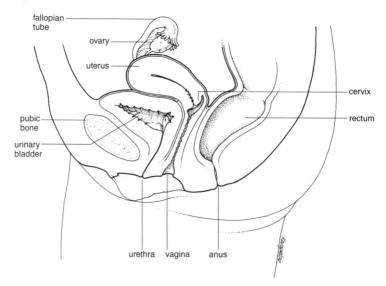

FIGURE 3 FEMALE SEX ORGANS

sullen, depressed, even irritable. The sight of the exquisite sleeping child did nothing to elevate her mood. She felt worn out, sloppy, ugly; she let her hair hang limp, not having the energy to wash it. And the last thing she felt like doing was breastfeeding this baby. "There's something wrong with me," she told her husband. "This isn't normal." Her husband was running out of patience. "Snap out of it, Bec," he said. "This is all in your head."

Of course, John's wife and Rebecca's husband could be right: maybe their spouses' problems are in their head, maybe they simply are suffering from depression. But maybe and in these cases, it's highly likely— maybe John and Rebecca are victims of imbalances of their sex hormones, imbalances that have induced depression, lethargy, lack of sexual drive.

MEN, WOMEN and HORMONES

Men and women are different mainly because of their hormones. Even though the two genders are becoming more alike in recent years in areas such as career goals, grooming, and financial expectations, there are still basic physical and mental traits that stay very different. For instance, male sex hormones make a man more aggressive by nature than a woman, not more assertive, more aggressive. This, of course, can be changed to a large extent by the mental attitude, upbringing, and personality of the boy. But the physical effects of these hormones cannot be changed so easily. The fact that men develop heart disease as early as their thirties and forties whereas women do not follow suit until after menopause is all due to the protection against heart disease provided by the female sex hormones. On the other hand, the blood clots faster in men—no doubt a trait that evolved to prevent the male from dying easily of wounds sustained in battle.

Sex hormones begin to have an impact on the body as early as the eighth week of pregnancy, when the testes start producing testosterone in the male fetus, resulting in the development of male sex organs (Figure 2). If testosterone is not present in the fetus, female sex organs (Figure 3) will develop. The next time sex hormones have this great an influence on the body is during adolescence, where they affect the tremendous growth spurt and control the sexual development of the teenager.

SEX HORMONES DURING PREGNANCY, CHILDHOOD AND ADOLESCENCE

During the first half of pregnancy, the fetus has high levels of FSH (follicle stimulating hormone), LH (luteinizing hormone), and LHRH (luteinizing hormone releasing hormone). Around the time of birth, the hypothalamus becomes very sensitive to estrogen and testosterone and reduces the amount of LHRH it releases into the bloodstream. The sex organs become very insensitive to FSH and LH and produce only tiny amounts of estrogen and testosterone. Because of these mechanisms, babies have enough hormone to differentiate their sex but children do not have so much that they mature sexually right from birth.

When puberty approaches, around the age of 11 in girls and 13 in boys, the hypothalamus suddenly starts to produce and liberate increased amounts of LHRH. No one knows exactly what in the body causes this to happen, but it seems to be at least partly under the control of messages from the higher centers of the brain. The LHRH causes bursts of LH, and to a lesser extent, FSH, to be released from the pituitary during sleep, as well as smaller amounts to be released during the day. Around the same time, the hypothalamus becomes very sensitive to sex hormones and the gonadotropins (FSH and LH); the higher their blood levels, the higher the output of LHRH. This, in turn, causes an even greater production of FSH, LH, estrogen, and testosterone by the sex organs and the adrenal glands.

The effects of the raised estrogen levels in girls is to cause breast development (the first sign of hormonal changes), changes in sweat glands that causes the sweat to gain an odor, changes in the vagina and its secretions, and enlargement of the external genital organs. The androgens produced by the ovaries and adrenal glands in girls control the growth of pubic and underarm hair.

Testosterone levels in boys increase two years later, and cause the testes to enlarge and produce sperm (with the help of FSH); enlargement of the larynx (Adam's apple); deepening of the voice; enlargement of the penis, prostate and seminal vesicles (which produce the fluid sperm swim in), and the epididymis and vas deferens (the tubes that connect the testes to the penis); growth of body and facial hair; changes in the sweat glands that give the sweat an odor; and changes in behavior that make the male aggressive.

At the onset of puberty, growth hormone is also released from the pituitary in greater quantities, as we discussed in the last chapter. This release is totally independent of the sex hormones and growth can occur without sexual development, as when GH is secreted normally but for some reason sex hormones are not secreted. In girls, most growth occurs before the first period (called menarche). After menarche, growth slows down and when the girl starts ovulating (usually several months after her first period) and estrogen reaches its adult level, growth stops. In boys, the growth spurt lasts for an average of two extra years, which is a major reason why they are taller.

The actual composition of the body—the percentage of muscle, fat, or bone—changes equally in boys and girls throughout childhood, but with the onset of puberty such similarities end. Girls develop more fat, accounting for their broader hips, rounded buttocks, and rounded breasts. (The shape and size of these features is greatly influenced by heredity.) Boys develop more muscle, heavier bones, and less fat, accounting for the male's greater physical strength.

MENSTRUATION

The increasing body weight and body fat content seems to trigger the onset of menarche in girls. Most girls have their first period when their weight reaches 105 pounds. This may happen anywhere from eight to sixteen years of age. Very thin girls with very little body fat, such as ballet dancers and long distance runners, go into menarche later. This partly explains why young girls who are afraid of sex and of growing up develop anorexia nervosa at this point. When their body weight drops to a very low point, they no longer menstruate.

Before we discuss menstruation, it's best to take a look at and understand the workings of the female body (see Figure 3). A woman is born with undeveloped eggs in her ovaries. Once a month, one or two of these eggs mature and are passed down the fallopian tubes to the uterus, where a fertilized egg implants itself and develops into a fetus. Every month, under the influence of the hormones estrogen and pro-gesterone, the lining of the uterus thickens to prepare itself for this possible pregnancy. If an egg meets and fuses with a sperm (which has been ejaculated by the male into the vaginal canal, and has swum up through the cervix into the uterus) it will become fertilized and implanted into this uterine wall. However, if no pregnancy takes place, the lining loosens up and is shed through the vagina.

Menstruation is this monthly shedding of some of the tissue lining the uterus (called the endometrium). It occurs during the first five days of the monthly cycle, when estrogen and progesterone are at very low levels. At this time, the pituitary is prompted by these levels to secrete LH and FSH, which stimulate the ovaries to produce a new monthly cycle. FSH stimulates the development of a new follicle (a sac containing an egg) in the ovary, and LH stimulates the follicle to produce estrogen.

During days six to twelve of the cycle, LH continues to rise, resulting in an increasing estrogen level, causing further increases in LH. At the same time, the rising estrogen levels decrease FSH secretion, preventing more follicles from maturing (or else the woman would be continually releasing eggs). During days twelve and thirteen, estrogen levels reach a peak and then begin to decline, and progesterone starts to be produced. On day fourteen, LH levels surge, and within thirty-six hours of this rise, a follicle releases its egg (a process called ovulation). The egg passes to the uterus. If it encounters a sperm there, it may become fertilized. The egg casing (called a corpus luteum) remains in the ovary where it increases in size and produces progesterone, the hormone that thickens the lining of the uterus to make it ready for the implantation and development of a fertilized egg.

On days fifteen to twenty-seven of the cycle, progesterone continues to rise, and LH and FSH drop to their lowest levels. The progesterone peaks at the twenty-second day and by day twenty-seven has doubled the thickness of the endometrium and causes it to produce fats and glycogen. These will provide nourishment for the fetus should there be one. If there is no pregnancy, the corpus luteum shrinks and stops producing progesterone, and the endometrium is gradually broken down and excreted through the vagina. On day twenty-eight, the cycle starts again.

Although menstrual cycles can last anywhere from twenty to forty days, the one thing constant in all women is that ovulation occurs fourteen days before menstruation. If a woman has sexual intercourse at this time of the cycle, she has a greater chance of getting pregnant than at any other time, although fertilization can still certainly occur after this point, when the egg is traveling down to the uterus.

MENSTRUAL PROBLEMS

PREMENSTRUAL TENSION SYNDROME (PMS)

Few women reading this book don't know what PMS is by now, and even fewer have never suffered from at least some of its symptoms. PMS can be loosely defined as a group of symptoms experienced by many women that appear four to ten days before menstruation and abruptly disappear after menstruation begins.

Maggie was a mess before her period. Although she never missed work or made mistakes in her job, inside she was suffering silently. She would feel depressed, hostile, and anxious; she would suffer from wide mood swings throughout the day. She would almost obsessively seek out either sweet or salty foods—chocolate bars, cookies, pretzels, things in which she might not even usually be interested. Her breasts were tender and she was swollen up with water throughout her body. She felt as if her face was puffed out beyond her ears. Maggie was suffering from a bad case of PMS. The good news is: she sought help. Her doctor took the condition seriously and treated her using some sound dietary techniques and supplements.

No one is sure what causes PMS, but it is believed to be caused by too little progesterone or too much prolactin (the hormone produced by the pituitary that stimulates the breasts to produce milk). You can treat PMS following some simple guidelines:

- Increase your intake of complex carbohydrates (to prevent low blood sugar).
- Take a daily supplement of thirty milligrams of vitamin B6 (to prevent depression).
- Reduce your intake of coffee, tea, colas, chocolate, and other forms of caffeine (which exacerbates all the symptoms).
- Limit alcohol to one drink per day (also to prevent low blood sugar, among other harmful affects).
- Limit tobacco use (because nicotine exacerbates the breast symptoms). '
- Take up swimming (because it eases water retention in the body).

MENSTRUAL CRAMPS

When these are bad, they can be very bad, and a male partner may often not understand how uncomfortable they can be. Painful periods (a condition known as dysmenorrhea) are thought to be caused by a high level of the hormones called prostaglandins in the muscles of the uterus, causing them to contract violently. This could reduce the blood flow supplying the muscles in the uterus, reducing their oxygen supply, and causing the pain due to a lack of oxygen. The cramps can be treated by using one of a number of drugs, including ibuprofen, fenoprofen, mefenamic acid, and naproxen. If the cramps do not occur during menstruation, but only when the woman is ovulating, the most effective way to cure the problem is to take birth control pills, which prevent ovulation.

ENDOMETRIOSIS

Either when a female child is first developing, or during menstruation, some cells from the lining of the uterus may become displaced to other areas of the body such as the fallopian tubes, the abdomen, the colon, outside the uterus, or even as far away as the lungs. This tissue responds to the sex hormones in the same ways as the lining of the uterus, and so each month it increases in size, bleeds, and attempts to break free into the menstrual flow. However, there is nowhere for this tissue to go and so it scars over. When this happens over a period of years, the scar tissue builds up and causes pressure in the organs, resulting in pain and heavier monthly bleeding. Sometimes the tissue has to be removed surgically, but it can often be treated instead with either birth control pills on a continuous basis rather than for just twenty-one days of the month, large doses of progesterone-like drugs, or male sex hormones.

HORMONAL BIRTH CONTROL

Almost one-third (29 percent) of American couples that practice birth control use oral contraceptives. They come in two basic types. The first is the combination pill, which contains synthetic estrogen and progesterone (called progestogen). This interferes with a woman's monthly hormonal fluctuations and prevents an egg from maturing and being released. The second type is called the mini-pill and it only contains progestogen. It does not prevent ovulation, but rather alters the lining of the uterus and the secretions keeping it moist so that neither the egg nor the sperm can survive within it.

Various side effects are experienced by women taking the pill. Those with a high estrogen content tend to cause migraine headaches, dark butterfly-shaped blotches on the face (called cholasma, also seen in pregnancy), breast tenderness and swelling, nausea, and weight gain. These problems may be corrected by switching to a lower estrogen pill or a mini-pill. Acne is sometimes caused by particular types of progestogens, and this can go away in a month or two when the woman is switched to a pill with a different type of progestogen or a higher estrogen content. Breakthrough bleeding (staining at other times of the month than menstruation) is more common on the mini-pill. The general rule here is that if the bleeding is in the early part of the cycle more estrogen is needed, but if it is during the latter part of the cycle more progestogen is required.

Several other kinds of pills have been developed. Two of these fall under the category of "morning-after pills." One contains a large dose of a type of estrogen called DES (diethylstilbestrol), which, if given within a day or two of intercourse, will change the lining of the uterus and prevent the implantation of a fertilized egg. This pill has not proved too successful so far because it has had such unpleasant side effects as nausea and vomiting, menstrual irregularities, and severe breast tenderness. DES was also used to prevent miscarriage until the early 1970s and led to an increased cancer risk in the daughters and possibly sons of the women who used it. It may also lead to breast cancer if taken regularly. However, DES is now sometimes administered only on a one-time basis and has mainly been used on women who must be quickly relieved of the developing fetus, such as rape victims.

The other kind of after-the-event pill has recently been created by French scientists and is called RU 486. This pill is taken once a month and blocks the action of progesterone, thereby preventing the implantation of the fertilized egg. If a woman is pregnant when she takes this pill, it brings on a menstrual period, terminating the pregnancy.

Some women use an IUD (intrauterine device) that releases small amounts of progesterone directly into the uterus, preventing implantation of the fertilized egg. IUDs are not as effective as oral contraceptives. The main negative side effect is that they can sometimes lead to high risk pregnancies: 50 percent of women who get pregnant using this device miscarry, have premature or still births, and run a greater risk of infection. The women may end up with a tubal pregnancy where the egg becomes implanted in the fallopian tubes and this can be life-threatening to the mother and/or damage her fallopian tubes so much that they can no longer convey eggs from the ovaries to the uterus.

THE PILL FOR MEN

Finally, in recent years, researchers have been working on an oral contraceptive for men. A hormone called inhibin which is present in men and thought to block the secretions of FSH (which in the male stimulates the testes to produce sperm), is now being tested. However, it still remains to be seen whether or not inhibin will prevent the formation of all sperm. This must be confirmed before it can be used as a form of birth control for one simple reason: whereas a 95 percent reduction in ovulation makes a woman virtually sterile, a man with only 5 percent of his normal sperm count will be almost as fertile as ever.

THE HORMONAL CHANGES OF PREGNANCY

Major hormonal changes are needed during pregnancy to prepare the mother's body for the growing fetus and to ensure normal fetal development. The thyroid gland enlarges and makes more thyroid hormone, which enhances the mother's ability to provide the extra energy needed by both her and the fetus. The adrenal glands increase their output: increased cortisol helps to boost the amount of energy available for new growth; increased aldosterone causes the body to retain more sodium and water in order to offset the sodium losses caused by the extra progesterone released during this time.

The placenta produces large amounts of estrogen, progesterone, human chorionic gonadotropin, ACTH, and human placental lactogen. These hormones help the fetus get all the nutrients it needs for optimal growth. The effects of all these changes in the mother's body are shown in Table 5.

TABLE 5

Hormonal Effects on the Mother's Body During Pregnancy

Gums become softer and bleed more readily
Hair grows thicker and faster, but large amounts may fall out within a
few months after delivery
The vagina becomes more susceptible to infection
Bowel habits change; the woman may develop diarrhea, constipation,
or a combination of the two
Frequent urination, to the point where some women even have blad-
der control problems
Hands and feet swell
Sinuses become congested
Cramps occur in the legs
Feelings of euphoria develop only to turn into depression after deliv-
ery when estrogen levels drop sharply (called postnatal depression)
Insomnia
Periods of high energy alternating with periods of extreme fatigue
Increased sensitivity of the skin to the sun; people who normally tan
will get a deep tan, and fair-skinned people will burn more easily
Moles and freckles become darker
The areola (area surrounding the nipple) becomes larger and darker
in color
A dark line may develop, going from the navel to the pubic hair re-
gion (called the linea nigra)
Dark, butterfly-shaped blotches may develop on the face and can be-
come darker upon exposure to the sun (called cholasma, or the
mask of pregnancy)
Blood volume increases

**Note: All of these changes usually reverse themselves within a few months
after delivery.**

GESTATIONAL DIABETES

Gestational diabetes is one of the most common complications of
pregnancy and affects between two and four percent of all pregnant
women in the United States. When it occurs, blood sugar levels shoot
up very high and only return to normal after the baby is born. Women
who suffer from this problem usually have a genetic predisposition to
diabetes mellitus (see the Guide) and the stress of pregnancy simply
brings on the disorder.

The mechanism that causes this condition is fairly clear. Because a pregnant woman needs so much more energy than the rest of us, she needs to produce more insulin to enable the cells of her body to absorb the energy they need. To complicate matters even more, estrogen, progesterone, and placental lactogen all work against the actions of insulin, and so even greater amounts are needed to overcome this effect. Also, raised cortisol levels make the liver release more glucose. Women who are genetically susceptible to diabetes may not be able to increase their production of insulin enough to satisfy these increased needs.

Gestational diabetes can threaten the life of the fetus and so all women receiving prenatal care are monitored for blood glucose levels throughout their pregnancies. Expectant mothers with this disorder are first placed on a special diet designed to normalize blood sugar levels. If this does not work, they are treated with insulin. Perhaps as many as half of all women who develop gestational diabetes will go on to develop non-insulin-dependent diabetes in later life.

HORMONAL INFLUENCES ON LABOR AND DELIVERY

No one is sure what exactly starts labor but all agree that it has something to do with a group of hormones called prostaglandins. The stepped-up production of prostaglandins that increase contractions in the uterus and soften the cervix could be due to hormones secreted by the fetus; the stretching of the uterus caused by the fetus; hormonal changes in the mother; or by milder contractions of the uterus. Once contractions have started, the hormone oxytocin, coming from the mother's pituitary, further promotes and sustains labor.

HORMONAL CHANGES AFTER DELIVERY

After a women gives birth, her hormonal state is very similar to what it is at menopause. She has hot flashes, perspires a great deal, suffers from irritability and mood swings, and is very depressed. This last symptom, called postnatal depression, can be quite serious. Remember Rebecca from the beginning of this chapter? She was suffering from postnatal depression and was literally a victim of her hormones. If a new mother shows signs of this condition, family members should be on the lookout for any warning signs that indicate she might need professional help. Some mothers have been so depressed after delivery they have done harm to their children or to themselves.

Why does such a severe depression appear during what should be a joyous time? Large quantities of hormones produced by the placenta during pregnancy raise the mother's blood levels, which in turn stop the production of similar hormones by the pituitary and ovaries. These endocrine glands are effectively turned off. However, it takes three to four months after delivery for these glands to start working normally again, and without the placental boost, there is nothing there to fill the gap.

Other hormonal changes occur after delivery. If a woman does not breastfeed her child she will get her period again in three to four months. If she does nurse the child, the hormone prolactin, which stimulates the breasts to produce milk, will delay the period for about six months. Oxytocin is also secreted by the pituitary at this time, to help the body conserve the salt and water needed for milk production.

CHANGE OF LIFE: THE MENOPAUSE

Menopause occurs when a woman stops ovulating and menstruation ceases. On average, this happens at around the age of fifty-one in most American women, although the ovaries function more and more slowly over a five to ten year period before the actual event.

A woman is born with two million immature eggs and by puberty is left with about three hundred thousand (the rest have withered and died). Thereafter, one or two will mature and others will die during the course of each menstrual cycle. By the time she reaches menopause, she will have perhaps as few as eight thousand remaining.

During the years right before menopause, the ovaries gradually decline in function. Periods become irregular and ovulation occurs infrequently. Sometimes two periods will come at almost the same time, only two to three weeks apart, and then there will be none for seven to eight weeks. When periods do come they are lighter and more watery with fewer clot-like substances. In some women, there is a heavy flow for one or two days, followed by several days without bleeding, and then several days of thin spotting. Eventually ovarian function declines even further and the periods stop completely. When a woman has been without a period for a year it usually means that menopause is complete.

However, women going into menopause must still be careful about birth control.

Sheila, a forty-eight-year-old high school teacher, had two children in college. She and her husband were struggling to pay a mountain of bills, both for their home as well as for college tuition. The last thing they planned on was another child. And Sheila didn't think there was much chance of that, since she was "around that age" and hadn't menstruated for over seven months. So she stopped using any form of birth control. A few months later, she began to feel nauseous and dizzy in the morning. Could it be a case of flu? She checked with her doctor and the news she heard was shocking! She was pregnant. Sheila discussed the situation with Bill, and they decided to have the child. Although they are now very happy with their young son, their two older children have had to switch to less expensive schools and are not totally thrilled with the situation. However, Sheila and Bill feel quite lucky. Sheila had tests done before their new son was born to verify his health. He was born normal, a healthy boy for two rather dazed older parents!

Older women run a much greater risk of having a child with some sort of birth defect than younger women do. Therefore prenatal testing of the fetus is recommended for older women. Without the proper tests before birth, older parents may be left with a child that is unexpected and unhealthy.

What happens during menopause? As the ovaries stop functioning they no longer produce estrogen. When this blood level goes down the pituitary responds by pushing out more and more LH and FSH in a futile attempt to get the ovaries going again. These changing hormonal levels can cause a number of symptoms, although some women do not experience any side effects from menopause.

HOT FLASHES (OR FLUSHES)

Three out of four menopausal women do suffer from hot flashes. These can be described as sudden rushes of heat that start in the chest and race upward to the arms, neck, and face. The skin flushes, the heart beats faster, breathing becomes more shallow, and sometimes the areas affected start to itch. As the hot flash passes (usually after a few minutes), the woman perspires and then feels cold and tired. Anything that affects the temperature of the body, such as exercise or entering a cold place, can bring on a hot flash. They also may occur spontaneously, a few times a day or several times an hour, and can continue in some women for months or even years. If they come on at night, they take the form of night sweats, which can cause insomnia.

VAGINAL SYMPTOMS

Several years after menopause, most women experience some vaginal burning and itching. When estrogen levels drop, the lips of the vagina and the vagina itself shrink, its lining becomes very thin, and its secretions diminish and become less acidic (making it prone to infection and making intercourse painful). These symptoms are much less severe in women who have sex frequently (three or more times a week) and have an orgasm (at least once a week).

OTHER PROBLEMS

Many women suffer from one or more of the following menopausal effects:

- Increased susceptibility to cystitis
- Palpitations
- Mood swings
- Fluid and weight gain around the stomach
- Increased or decreased interest in sex
- Breasts that are less lumpy, softer, and have less elasticity, causing sagging.

Women who have hysterectomies often experience worse symptoms than women who go through menopause naturally. However, you should know that all of the symptoms mentioned can be successfully treated with estrogen, which can also protect women against osteoporosis (by preventing bone loss), heart disease (by preventing the rise in blood cholesterol that accompanies menopause), and rheumatoid arthritis (by suppressing any possible inflammation of the joints).

There are drawbacks to giving estrogen on its own. It causes a thickening of the lining of the uterus and so causes an increased risk of cancer. For this reason, hormone replacement therapy usually involves giving both estrogen and progesterone. Estrogen is taken for twenty days, then progesterone and estrogen are taken together for ten days, and finally nothing is taken for the next five days, and so on. This allows the uterine lining to be shed (as it is during the menstrual period) and while it causes a light period, it negates the increased risk of cancer. Progesterone also protects the breasts against cancer. During the first two or three months on this type of therapy, a woman may suffer from nausea, weight gain, swollen breasts, headaches, dizziness, vaginal infections, and breakthrough bleeding, but these usually pass with time.

THE TRUTH ABOUT MALE MENOPAUSE

While there is no formal male menopause, the same way there is in women, men's bodies do change as they get older. When men reach their sixties or seventies (possibly even a bit earlier) their testes produce smaller and smaller amounts of testosterone, which can make them less interested in sex (although this is certainly not a rule), less fertile, and sometimes even impotent. They may become depressed and lethargic. If you recall John from the beginning of the chapter you'll get a picture of what this hormonal change is like. Hormone replacement therapy can help these conditions but unfortunately it is associated with an increased risk of heart disease and strokes (because it raises cholesterol levels), and prostate cancer.

Over a lifetime, the testosterone in a man's body causes his prostate to grow and partially block the urethra, through which urine flows from the bladder to the outside. Some men develop cancer of the prostate, but at such an advanced age that it is said the majority of men die with it but few die of it. However, testosterone therapy could speed up the development of this disease.

If prostate cancer is caught early enough it can be treated by completely removing the gland using a surgical procedure called a prostatectomy. However, this type of cancer can spread to the lower part of the spine, the pelvis, and the hips, causing bone pain. By lowering testosterone levels in the body, you can stop the areas to which it has spread from getting any bigger and even cause them to shrink for a year or more. This may be done by either removing the testes or by giving drugs such as cyproterone that prevent the production of androgen in the testes and adrenal glands. Alternatively, estrogens, which have a similar effect, may be given, although they tend to cause the development of feminine traits (such as the growth of breasts). If the areas of the bone where the cancer has spread do not respond to hormone therapy, they are treated with radiotherapy.

HORMONES AND OTHER PROBLEMS: IMPOTENCE, INFERTILITY . . .

You've probably seen talk shows about impotence or heard of couples trying every possible measure to overcome infertility. For a more detailed discussion of these and other problems caused by imbalances of the sex hormones, see the Guide.

HOW HORMONES AFFECT THE BREAST

The breasts are extremely sensitive to changes in estrogen, prolactin, and oxytocin levels in a woman's body. Even in the womb, these hormones may pass across the placenta to the unborn baby and cause some breast tissue to develop in both boys and girls. However, right after birth these hormones are shed from the infant's body and the breast tissue shrinks until adolescence, when a rise in estrogen levels in girls once again causes breast development, this time for good.

DURING PREGNANCY AND LACTATION

The first sign of pregnancy is a change in the size and shape of the breasts, around the time of the first missed period. The breasts become swollen and tender and the areola surrounding the nipple becomes larger and darker in color. After the first few weeks the tenderness subsides but the breasts continue to become fuller due to the influence of rising sex hormone levels. During the last half of pregnancy, thin milky fluids and sometimes a drop of blood may be discharged from the breasts. Just before giving birth the breasts become very engorged and these discharges may increase in volume and frequency.

When the baby sucks on the nipple, the mother's pituitary gland produces prolactin, which stimulates the breasts to produce milk and oxytocin, which causes the breasts to eject the milk through the nipples. The breasts will continue to produce milk as long as the child sucks on them. Other stimuli can also make the breasts of a new mother secrete milk, such as the cry of a baby or sexual arousal.

COMPOSITION, MENSTRUATION AND FIBROCYSTIC DISEASE

Breasts are made up of glandular tissue that produces milk and fat tissue. This gives them their characteristic shape. They are supported by ligaments and skin. Both their size and composition is changed by the rise and fall of hormonal levels during the menstrual cycle. High levels of progesterone and estrogen in the premenstrual phase increase blood flow to the breasts, promote water retention which makes the breasts swell, and stimulate the growth of the glandular tissue. When the hormonal levels go down during menstruation, the swelling goes down as the water and extra glandular tissue is slowly reabsorbed. However, before this can be fully done, the next menstrual cycle begins, and once again rising hormonal levels stimulate fluid retention and the growth of more glandular tissue. Over a period of years, this extra tissue and fluid forms fibrocysts (essentially fluid-filled sacs).

When she was in her twenties, Martha discovered fitness and really got her life on track. She was bound and determined to move into her thirties maintaining all these good habits. She wouldn't have to age. And it's true that when she turned thirty she didn't feel suddenly old, or fatigued, or unattractive. Not at all. But she did notice a few signs that her body was changing. And one of the strangest was that her breasts seemed to be changing in composition. They were lumpy. Though anxious, she sensibly went immediately to her physician for tests for breast cancer. But Martha was lucky. She tested negative. "So what's wrong with my breasts?" she asked her doctor. Her physician explained that she had simply developed fibrocysts and that this was quite a common occurence.

Most women by the age of thirty have lumpy breasts because of the formation of fibrocysts. The older a woman becomes, the worse they tend to get, up until menopause, when the lumpiness begins to subside.

You can take the following steps to ease the condition:

- Avoid beverages with a high caffeine content;
- Avoid salt or salty foods;
- Wear a brassiere at all times, even a light one to bed;
- Try a supplement of 400-800 IUs of vitamin E daily (which seems to help some women).

In addition, your physician might try a number of different methods to treat fibrocystic disease including:

- Birth control pills (which help some women and make others worse);
- An antiestrogen drug such as tamoxifen;
- Draining the fibrocysts.

AN IMPORTANT NOTE: Remember that not all breast lumps are tumors, but not all are fibrocysts either. If you note any changes in your breasts, or if you detect a lump, consult your physician immediately. Breast cancer strikes too many women for you to take chances. See the following section.

BREAST CANCER

One out of eleven American women develop breast cancer at some time during the course of life. Two out of three breast tumors seem to be stimulated by either estrogen, progesterone, or prolactin. Such tumors are usually treated with surgery but the manipulation of hormone levels can be beneficial in about one-third of all cases. For instance, premenopausal women are often treated with antiestrogen drugs such as tamoxifen to reduce their estrogen levels. Aminoglutethimide is another drug used, and it works by preventing the adrenals from producing androgens. Androgens are converted to estrogen in fat tissue, which might be the reason why breast cancer is most commonly found in obese women. Sometimes the cancer is treated by taking prolactin out of the body through the surgical removal of the pituitary gland. When the disease is advanced and antiestrogen drugs have not worked, the administration of progesterone often results in some improvement. As an alternative, hormone therapy can be used in conjunction with chemotherapy, and this often yields quicker results.

YOUR HORMONES AND SEXUAL RELATIONSHIPS

We are now discovering that a substance produced by the body, called a pheromone, may play a major role in the attraction between the sexes and the timing of the woman's monthly cycle. The substances known as pheromones, discovered thirty years ago, are thought to be found throughout the animal kingdom. They are secreted by female dogs when they are in heat, attracting all the male dogs within sniffing distance. Their release may attract male butterflies to the females that are ready to mate. Now it turns out that they could play a big role in human sexuality as well. So you thought it was his eyes, or her body that turned you on? Guess again, it's probably those pheromones! For more on this fascinating subject, see the next chapter.

IN CONCLUSION

Throughout our lives, sex hormones have a tremendous influence on our bodies and behavior. They play a major role in growth, emotions, susceptibility to disease, and the aging process. Their importance has often been missed in the past, when conditions such as PMS, menopause, infertility, and impotence were thought of as "just the way it is," or "part of getting older," mainly because these problems were not life-threatening. However, as we learn more about the way sex hormones work in our bodies, we can see that all these disorders will become treatable.

Perhaps the most amazing piece of news came as we were writing this book: in the future, through the manipulation of sex hormones, and the implantation of a fertilized egg into the abdomen, a man may be able to become pregnant and carry a baby to term!

CHAPTER SEVEN

BEHAVIOR, PERSONALITY AND RELATIONSHIPS

Bridget was divorcing Bob, her husband of ten years, so she wasn't terribly surprised when she started to feel anxious and upset upon awakening in the morning. She grew worried, however, when these anxiety attacks became more frequent and stronger, coming upon her at all times of the day. She went to see a psychiatrist. The doctor also assumed the problem was stemming from her divorce proceedings and prescribed an antidepressant.

After two weeks of more anxiety and no relief coming from the medication, Bridget felt like committing herself to an institution. Her nervousness was now even making her hair fall out; her skin began to feel thin and bruised. She was not eating properly either, but was surprised to see she had lost over twenty pounds.

One night, Bridget's best friend Virginia invited her to a dinner party. Over the meal, someone mentioned how traumatic divorce was; Bridget laughingly said that it was not only making her thin and anxious, it was also thinning out her skin and hair. One of the other guests, a young woman, asked her to elaborate, and Bridget shyly told her the symptoms she had been suffering from. The young woman then introduced herself as a doctor. She asked Bridget to come down to her office for a few tests. Bridget did, and these tests revealed what the doctor had first suspected; that Bridget was not suffering from a psychiatric disorder, but rather a hormonal one. Her thyroid gland was overworking, giving her the symptoms of thinning hair, thin skin, excessive weight loss, and anxiety. After treatment, all of Bridget's symptoms disappeared.

In a way, Bridget was lucky. Along with her mood problems, other physical symptoms appeared. People with hormonal problems sometimes only have the psychological symptoms and are frequently mistaken for psychiatric patients. What is important for you to understand from all this is that your hormones don't only run your brain and body to a large extent, they also exert a tremendous influence on your behavior, mood, and relationships.

It has been known for some time that the male hormone testosterone is responsible for a man's aggressive tendencies. However, it has recently come to light that other hormones have just as powerful an effect on such traits as shyness, the ability to cope with stress, mental illness, and the attraction between men and women.

MALES AND TESTOSTERONE

Even though there are more men than women born in the industrialized world, when the old people gather, there are mainly women in the crowd. This is because women outlive men by anywhere from four to ten years. Fifteen percent more males are conceived than females, and five percent more males than females are born. However, equal numbers of both sexes are around by age thirty, and only 70 percent of men reach age sixty-five, whereas 84 percent of women do.

In the latter half of life, cardiovascular disease accounts for most of this gap. The female hormone estrogen protects women from the disease up until menopause, and few have developed bad enough heart disease to kill them at age sixty-five. On the other hand, men's arteries have been suffering from blockages since the cradle.

Homicide also accounts for many more male deaths, especially in the first half of life. In fact, one study showed that four times as many men are killed than women. Obviously, many of those murdered were engaged in violent crimes or businesses at the time of their demise. This violent tendency on the part of the male, which seems to be for the most part absent in the female, is probably due to the influence of testosterone, which increases aggressive tendencies. (Of course, there are always exceptions, and there are violent women, but this could be due more to environment, opportunity, drug addiction or other forms of mental illness.) Studies show that men convicted of violent crimes very often have higher than average male hormone levels. It is also probably more than a coincidence that men are most likely to commit such crimes from the ages of sixteen to eighteen, when testosterone levels are at their peak. Naturally, most men do not chose to channel aggressiveness into violent acts, but the possibility may be there in their hormonal systems.

As well as influencing aggression testosterone also increases the sex drive. Male sex offenders who have been found guilty of exhibitionism, rape, and child molestation often have high testosterone levels. And it is not unheard of for a judge to give the offender the opportunity to take cyproterone acetate, a drug that blocks the action of testosterone, instead of serving a lengthy jail sentence. This drug often controls the deviant behavior and lets the less violent of these men function normally in society.

POSITIVES AND NEGATIVES OF CORTISOL

When we are under stress, our adrenal glands push out a great deal of cortisol. This hormone then enables us to stand up to the boss, remain alert when walking down that dark alley, or be a little bit sharper when we have to take an exam. But it has a lot of negative effects, as well. Patients with Cushing's disease (the excess production of cortisol—see the Guide) are profoundly depressed. In fact, many suicidal patients and manic depressives are found to have high cortisol levels. (Some manic patients also seem to be influenced by their hormones: they have been found to have high thyroxine and norepinephrine levels and low testosterone levels.)

Children who are very shy sometimes have higher cortisol levels than more extroverted children, and children who mature late and find it difficult to accept growing up also appear to have too much cortisol in operation.

When we are under stress, or warned about something, cortisol affects us in other ways. We lose our sex drives, cannot sleep well, and lose our appetites. If this stress persists over a long period of time its effects can be serious, even life-threatening. While the stress of an exam can sharpen the student's mind temporarily by bringing more oxygen and nutrients to the brain, worrying throughout the year about exams can make the same student more susceptible to infections, especially respiratory ones, since cortisol reduces the activity of the immune system. The same problem crops up in grieving people, who often become ill.

Kurt was a forty-year-old man who lost his wife to cancer. Since he was devoted to her, he found it hard to get on with his life even after she had been gone for over a year. He then started to come down with one illness after another and finally suffered from a respiratory infection that become so severe he had to be hospitalized. His family doctor advised Kurt to see an analyst, who over time helped him to cope with his wife's absence. Five years later, Kurt remarried. Although he will never totally forget his first wife, his health is back to normal again.

Cortisol may also make a preexisting mental illness even worse. For instance, stress can speed up the progression of Alzheimer's disease. All in all, stress, through the cortisol it causes to be released, can have far-reaching effects on your state of mind and body, and unfortunately, a lot of it is bad. Drugs are now being developed to block the production of CRH and hence the production of ACTH and cortisol, in order to help relieve stress.

ENDORPHINS

Endorphins and enkephalins, compounds produced by the brain, both have profound effects on our everyday performance. They are the natural morphine of the body and as such are responsible for modulating pain, causing the "runner's high," for example. Some chronic pain sufferers are fitted with an electrical device that stimulates the brain to secrete endorphins and thereby provide relief. Also, lately endorphins have been implicated in PMS and a psychiatric problem known as post traumatic stress disorder (PTSD).

When you take a drug away from an addict, he or she experiences withdrawal. One theory now suggests that a similar phenomenon explains PMS. Women with this disorder may have an abnormal sensitivity to endorphins. When their levels decline, just before menstruation, a withdrawal-type reaction could occur.

Post-traumatic stress disorder (PTSD) affects survivors of battles, crashes, earthquakes, and other nightmarish experiences. The survivors of the Nazi death camps, as well as Vietnam veterans, are two large groups who often suffer from this disorder. Months or years after the event, these people believe the experience is happening again, and again. They may have terrifying nightmares and extreme emotional distress. PTSD can disrupt a person's whole life. Recently, it has been discovered that these "flashbacks" are accompanied by massive out-pourings of endorphins. If this can be confirmed, then perhaps drugs like naloxone, that block the actions of endorphins, may be used to help people with this problem.

GROWTH HORMONE AND SUICIDE

Suicide is a major problem in our society. There were 29,453 suicides in this country in 1985, and 2,127 of them were teenagers. New data shows that many adolescents who attempt to commit suicide have lower growth hormone levels than teenagers who are depressed but do not try to kill themselves. Further research should shed more light on this possible link.

OXYTOCIN AND MATERNAL INSTINCTS

Oxytocin is thought to be involved in what is known as the "mater-nal instincts." In animals, it stimulates a mother to lick and caress her offspring. It may also explain why some women respond more than men do to a baby's cry.

PHEROMONES

Pheromones are the name given to hormonal substances which, when released by one person, cause changes in the behavior or physical state of another. Their presence and release might explain why some people get along with one another and others do not. It could be that you only enjoy people who release a certain type of pheromone.

These substances could figure into life right from the beginning. A baby may be attracted to his mother's breast because of her pheromones. Roommates at college often find that their menstrual cycles move closer together until eventually they begin menstruation at the exact same time. This phenomenon has recently been shown to be possibly caused by pheromonal action. In an experiment, some underarm perspiration from one woman was placed on the upper lip of other women three times a week for three months. At the start of the experiment, all the women were menstruating at individual times. But after three months of this "treatment" the women began to menstruate at about the same time as the woman who donated the perspiration.

How do pheromones affect sexual relationships? Well, one way to examine this was to repeat the same kind of experiments, this time using men and women. Male underarm sweat was placed on the upper lips of seven women three times a week. At the beginning of the study, the women had menstrual cycles of varying lengths, ranging from 26 days to 33 days. By the end of the third month, the women all had cycles of exactly 29.5 days, which is the optimal cycle length for conception. Thus, male sweat contained something that altered the women's reproductive cycle to make them more likely to become pregnant.

Although these experiments have been severely criticized, many people agree that sweat does contain substances that affect our behavior in subtle ways. Some feel that these pheromones are actually a compound called androstenol (similar to androgens) and the compound's levels change in a woman's sweat in a cyclic way, so as to peak just before ovulation. Perhaps this was an adaptation from our animal heritage, when there were more convenient times than others to mate and all the females had to be "ready" at once.

In the beginning of all this speculation, there came a story from a scientist who maintained that when he was marooned on a desert island without any female company his beard grew more slowly, due to a lack of female "essence." Since then, we have tried many experiments to find out the importance and validity of pheromones. We still have a long way to go. Even the strongest supporters of pheromonal theory think that they affect human behavior only in the subtlest of ways.

HORMONES AND EMOTIONS

Remember Bridget, the anxious woman in the beginning of the chapter? Well, as you will see from the guide section of this book, most hormonal diseases are accompanied by behavioral signs and symptoms, mainly anxiety and/or depression. Clearly, our hormonal balance is crucial to our state of mind and any changes in that balance, whether they are caused by endocrine diseases or self-imposed by conditions like stress, can radically alter our mood, behavior, and personality.

THE COSMETIC ANGLE: YOUR SKIN AND HAIR

Paula had always been proud of her flawless complexion. Both she and her mother enjoyed clear, creamy skin, with never even a hint of a pimple. After Paula and her husband had their two children, she decided to go on birth control pills. About two months after starting the pills, Paula's skin changed drastically. It became oily and spotted, almost as though she was suffering from adolescent acne. At first she thought it might be her diet or something in the air. But as her skin condition got worse, she sought help from her physician. He explained that certain types of progesterone found in birth control pills can lead to skin problems, even in women who had never before suffered from them. He switched her pill and within several months Paula's skin went right back to normal.

Hormones have a strong impact on your skin and hair. Hormonal diseases can change the look and nature of your skin and cause your hair to become limp and dry, or even to fall out. Sometimes they are the first or only signs of a serious hormonal imbalance. So, should either your hair or your skin change suddenly, it is best to see your physician immediately and take the appropriate tests.

Your skin is the largest organ of your body. It is much more than a simple covering to protect the body from wear and tear and infections. It produces and activates hormones, enzymes, and other substances that have important roles in the body. This is why losing vast amounts of skin the way burn victims do can be life-threatening. Hair is derived from the skin and is mostly dead tissue. But it can still indicate the presence of disease. Keeping a careful eye on the state of your outside can often protect and correct the inside.

YOUR SKIN

The skin is made up of two layers, the epidermis is the outside one, and the dermis is right underneath it. Five percent of the cells in the epidermis are melanocytes and produce the pigment melanin, which gives your skin its color and protects it from the harmful ultraviolet rays of the sun. The other 95 percent are called keratinocytes and produce a number of substances crucial to the body, such as:

- vitamin D
- T3, produced from T4 (the thyroid hormones)
- interferons, that kill viruses
- interleukins, integral parts of the immune system
- collagenase, which helps prevent wrinkles
- apolipoprotein E, that helps the body break down cholesterol
- thymopoietin, which stimulates the body to make T-lymphocytes that help fight infections
- a host of hormone-like substances currently being investigated
- nails
- hair

Keratinocytes manufacture a protein called keratin which gives the skin its resilience. The keratinocytes are in various stages of development or deterioration. The cells on the surface are dead and continuously being shed, whereas the underlying cells are actively producing the crucial substances listed above. The whole of the epidermis is replaced every fifteen to thirty days.

The dermis is much thicker and contains nerve endings, blood vessels, sebaceous glands (that help keep the skin supple and at times oily), sweat glands, hair follicles, and muscles. Underneath the dermis is a layer of fat that serves as an energy store and protects us from the cold. This fat also helps convert androgens (male hormones) to estrogens (female hormones) in women.

TABLE 6
Good Food Sources of Vitamins A and C

Vitamin A	Vitamin C
Apricots	Broccoli
Asparagus	Brussels sprouts
Beans (green)	Cantaloupe
Broccoli	Cauliflower
Brussels sprouts	Cranberry juice
Cantalope	Grapefruit juice
Carrots	Kale
Corn	Lemon juice
Eggs	Orange
Liver	Orange juice
Milk	Parsley
Orange juice	Papaya
Peaches	Peppers
Peas	Pineapple juice
Sweet potatoes	Spinach
Pumpkin	Strawberries
Squash	Collard greens
Tomato juice	Mustard greens
Yogurt	Turnip greens

HOW TO CARE FOR YOUR SKIN

Good skin care starts with good nutrition. What you put into your mouth is more important to the look of your complexion than what you put on top of it. The two most important nutrients for the skin are vitamins A and C (good sources are shown in Table 6). You should also drink plenty of water, about eight glasses daily, to keep the skin clear and moist.

As you get older the skin begins to lose some of its elasticity and dries out, leading to sagging, wrinkling, and cracking. Unfortunately, this is inevitable, because the sebaceous glands produce less sebum (oil), and that youthful glow starts to disappear. But other factors can influence how quickly and how well you age. Heredity has a lot to do with it. If your parents don't have many wrinkles then you probably won't either, unless you have indulged in a skin destroyer, such as smoking, drinking, or excess tanning.

If you live in a dry, sunny climate, like California, your skin is more likely to become leathery and wrinkled than in a damp, cloudy environment like England. As we just mentioned, smoking also causes more wrinkling. In women, this is thought to be partly due to the fact that smoking lowers estrogen levels and estrogen appears to increase sebum production. This is why women's skin feels softer than men's.

No over-the-counter creams or lotions can cause a lasting improvement in wrinkled skin, no matter what the advertisements say. The only treatment that seems to have some affect on wrinkles involves a medication called retinoic acid (Retin-A), and more research and time is needed before any conclusive statements can be made. There also appear to be some unpleasant side effects to Retin-A. One easy and positive thing you can do for aging skin is to rehydrate it, by soaking it with water and then immediately covering the wet face with petroleum jelly, moisturizer, or skin cream to prevent the water from evaporating.

SKIN AND HORMONES: ACNE

Three out of four people get acne at some time in their lives. Most boys and girls develop it during their adolescent years and many women suffer from it again at menopause. No one knows exactly what causes it but most agree that hormones are involved. Androgens are probably the biggest culprits, although changes in hormonal levels as during menstruation, pregnancy, stress, menopause, or the use of birth control pills can cause a flare-up.

Acne starts in the sebaceous glands, which secrete their sebum into the hair follicle. This sebum, consisting of cholesterol and dead cells, is pushed to the surface and liberated up through the follicle and onto the surface of the skin through the follicle openings (also called the pores of the skin). As the sebum does this, it lubricates the hair shaft.

The production of sebum is greatly increased at adolescence due to the action of androgens, which is why acne seldom appears before this time. The sebum, along with keratin and bacteria that live in the hair follicle, form a plug called a comedo, that blocks the follicle. When the follicle is blocked at the surface of the skin a whitehead is formed, from the white or skin-colored plug material. If the comedo protrudes further than the pore it becomes black in color (a blackhead) due to the presence of pigmented cells. Finally, if the buildup of material in the follicle is great enough to burst the follicle within the skin, the bacteria and its contents will be spread under the skin causing a localized infection that forms a puss-filled mound called a pimple.

Teenage boys have higher androgen levels than teenage girls and so more acne. People with oily skin and hair may have a worse problem, but this is not always true. Severe inflammatory acne, causing scarring, is certainly inherited. However, acne is not caused by diet, lack of sleep, sex (either too little or too much) or masturbation.

Mild acne can be treated by keeping the skin and hair free of oil with frequent washing (using a cloth to remove the outer layer of dead cells), and shampooing. Benzoyl peroxide, which removes dead cells from the surface of the skin, is also good. You can start with a five percent solution and build up to one with no more than ten percent. For more severe cases, antibiotics can be used, either as a cream rubbed into the skin or in pill form. Tetracycline or erythromycin are usually the ones prescribed for acne.

Finally, physicians also prescribe drugs made from vitamin A, which are taken orally. One of these is the same drug we mentioned earlier, retinoic acid or tretinoin (Retin-A), which causes the skin to peel (and may help wrinkling). The other, called isotretinoin (Accutane), prevents sebum production. However, both of these drugs may have unpleasant side effects and the patient must weigh the benefits against the liabilities.

Oral contraceptives containing estrogen can improve the situation, but the mini-pill (along with certain types of regular pills) can make the condition worse due to its progesterone content. Progesterone is the reason why acne gets worse in some women right before their periods: at this time, progesterone levels are high, which makes the hair follicle openings smaller and more likely to get clogged.

Finally, the use of too much makeup can also cause acne by blocking the pores.

THE SKIN AND HORMONAL DISEASES

Many hormonal disorders cause skin problems (see the Guide). If you suffer from a sudden change in your skin, the following illnesses could be to blame:

TABLE 7
Hormonal Problems That Affect Skin

Disorder	Skin Problem
Underactive thyroid	Thickened skin that is rough and dry.
Overactive thyroid	Thinning skin with increased sweating.
All thyroid disease	Vitiligo, or white patches of skin with no pigment on hands, face, arms, around skin folds and openings due to death of pigment cells, can be cured with drugs called psoralens, or by transplanting pigment cells from other parts of the body. Itching.
Addison's disease	Skin pigmentation changes; skin darkens and freckles can develop on forehead and upper body. Surroundings of nipples, mouth, lips, and vagina become bluish-black. Vitiligo.
Cushing's disease	Thinning skin that easily bruises. Purple stretch marks on the stomach.

YOUR HAIR

All over your body, except for the soles of your feet, the palms of your hands, the skin around your mouth, anus, and other openings to the outside of the body, you have hair. We have, in fact, just as many hair follicles as apes and chimpanzees but most of them produce vellus hairs, which are colorless and soft. Over the scalp, eyebrows, and eyelashes we produce terminal hair, which is much thicker. At puberty in a boy, rising testosterone levels convert the vellus hairs in the armpits, around the genitals, on the face, chest, arms and legs, to terminal hairs. Although women have as many hair follicles as men, the rising testosterone levels in their bodies at puberty only convert vellus into terminal hairs in the armpits and around the genitals, with perhaps a few of these hairs appearing on the upper lip, chin, around the nipples, and at various other spots.

Hairs are produced when cells in the root start to quickly multiply. As cells move up through and further away from the dermis they produce a protein called keratin which becomes harder the further away the cells move. The cells forming the hair change into two different types: there is a solid core of pigment-producing cells and an outer cuticle (skin) of scaly cells. All the cells forming the visible hair shaft are dead and only those at the root are alive.

HAIR GROWTH CYCLES

Hair grows in cycles. There is a growing or anagen phase when the cells at the bottom of the root are rapidly dividing and causing the hair to grow longer. This lasts from two to six years. Facial and scalp hair grows the fastest and longest, while the hair on top of the arm grows the slowest and lasts for the shortest amount of time. The second, or catagen phase, lasts for just a few weeks. The roots become filled with keratin, the blood supply to the root is reduced, and the root dies. The last is the resting or teleogen phase, when the old hair is shed as a new hair bulb forms at the bottom of the follicle. About one-third of your hairs are in each phase at any point in time. By the way, these phases are biological, and cutting the hair neither makes it grow faster nor slower.

In males and females, hair gets thinner with age, though in some men this thinning is pronounced. Baldness in men is caused by testosterone, provided that they have the genetic tendency toward the problem. In women total baldness or excessive thinning is very rare. However, after menopause, when estrogen levels are low, it is not uncommon to see women's hair get a little thinner on their heads and for them to grow some hairs on their faces.

CARING FOR YOUR HAIR

The hair shaft is covered in tightly overlapping cuticle cells covered by a thin coating of oil. Teasing, blow-drying, dyes, and permanents separate the layers of cuticle cells causing split ends, or at the very least swell the cells, making the surface of the hair uneven. As with many surfaces, the smoother it is, the more it shines, which is why hair damaged in this way becomes dull and dry. While conditioners can smooth out the cuticle cells and coat the hair with oil that makes it shine again, they cannot restore the hair permanently in any way.

Everyone's scalp flakes to some degree. Some begin flaking within twenty-four hours of being washed while with others it takes several days. Flaking, more commonly known as dandruff, can be prevented by frequent washing of the hair with a mild (nondetergent) shampoo, followed by thorough rinsing.

Your hair color is produced by melanocytes in the follicle that produce either melanin in brown- and black-haired people, or phaeomelanin in blonds, redheads, and people with auburn hair. Graying is caused by a gradual reduction in pigment production; when no pigment is made the hair turns white. There is still no way to prevent these telltale markers of time from appearing and increasing in number. You can throw out all the "special" vitamins, minerals, and synthetic creams and solutions that claim to stop your hair from turning gray; they don't work. But what might work is a hormone-like substance, currently being explored by researchers, that will stimulate aging melanocytes to produce greater quantities of pigment for a longer period of time. While this can't completely prevent the graying process, it may delay it.

THE HAIR AND HORMONAL DISEASES

Perhaps the most troublesome hair-related hormonal problem is a condition known as hirsutism (see the Guide). It can be caused by an excess of testosterone in women, due to a number of hormonal problems. As we mentioned, testosterone causes the fine vellus hairs to be converted into the pigmented and coarser terminal hairs.

Testosterone is carried in the blood both in a free form as well as bound to proteins called globulins. But it is only in its free state that it has any effect on the hair. Usually a mere one percent of all testosterone in the body is free, but women with hirsutism may have as much as two percent in this form. Estrogen increases the binding of testosterone to globulins and therefore lowers the level of these free culprits. When a woman goes into menopause and her estrogen levels drop, she develops more terminal hairs. Women who lose their periods due to excess physical training or dieting also tend to develop more terminal hair because of reduced estrogen levels. Other causes of the same problem include polycystic disease, ovarian cancer, adrenal gland disease, and the taking of certain drugs (androgens, cortisol, progesterone, phenytoin, and chlorpromazine). Unfortunately, even after the hormonal balance has been corrected, the excess hair that has already grown will remain. Electrolysis or some other hair removal method can be used.

HAIR LOSS

Rick was surprised when he started to lose his hair at the age of thirty. Many of his friends were already thinning out on the top and sides, but his father and grandfather both had full heads of hair. He became more and more disheartened each day as he picked hairs out of the sink, the bath, his brush, off the floor, and from his clothing. Finally Rick went to see his doctor, who took a series of endocrine tests. But every result was negative. Rick was fine. Then the doctor questioned Rick further and found out that he had recently started a new and very demanding job. Emotional stress, not genetics or disease, was to blame for Rick's hair loss. Stress increased Rick's androgen level, resulting in hair loss. Although Rick began to take it a bit easier by learning relaxation techniques, the hair he lost did not return. However, no more hair fell out once his stress level was reduced.

The most common hormonal cause of hair loss, besides the effects of androgens already mentioned, is thyroid disease. Bald patches can appear anywhere on the body where hair has grown. However, the loss is usually temporary and the hair grows back once the condition has been corrected. Thyroid disease can also cause premature (before the age of thirty) graying.

Abnormal hair loss can also be caused by any condition that forces all the hair into a resting phase such as a high fever, chemotherapy, X-ray therapy, the use of certain drugs, and withdrawal from birth control pills. As all the hairs are in the same phase they will all fall out at the same time. However, in many cases the hair will grow back. Hair may also be lost by pregnant women after they give birth due to the fall in estrogen levels, but this hair also normally returns.

IN CONCLUSION

The way our skin and hair look is very important to the way we feel about ourselves and so we should take special care of both. Any physical condition that endangers them can be psychologically devastating. In addition, the appearance and condition of the skin and hair can become early warning signs of various diseases, including hormonal ones.

CHAPTER NINE

THE FUTURE OF HORMONE RESEARCH

As we have seen, a lot is known about the role of hormones in the growth and development of the body as well as in the maintenance of mental and physical health. But there is still a lot left to know and a great deal of ongoing research being done in this area. In fact, hormones may hold the key to longevity itself. We already understand that one of the major components of a healthy body and mind is the proper hormonal balance. Excesses or deficiencies in certain hormones can lead to disease and even a shortening of the life span (see the Guide). Therefore, it only stands to reason that by learning more about hormones and the way they work we may one day be able to maintain a perfect balance in the body at all times and possibly prolong life beyond the seventy or eighty year expectancy we now enjoy. In this chapter, we will look at how several different fields of research are uncovering the importance and impact of hormones on our everyday lives and where this information might lead.

THE TOUCH OF DEVELOPMENT

New research has uncovered the fact that a mother's touch actually stimulates the growth of her children. Pediatricians have long noticed that premature babies who were fed intravenously and kept in incubators grew more slowly than similar babies who were picked up and held from time to time. Recently, scientists have been studying a similar phenomenon in animals. When baby rats are kept away from their mothers even for a period of forty-five minutes their metabolism starts to slow down. This is good in one sense: a slower metabolism means that the rat requires less energy, which would be needed for its possible survival if the mother was not around to feed it. On the other hand, if this happens frequently enough, the rat will grow more slowly.

Through these experiments, it was discovered that contact with the mother reduces the release of endorphins. Endorphins normally reduce the levels of growth hormone and insulin in the child's body, which stimulate growth. Hence, premature infants isolated from their mothers may have higher endorphin levels and therefore lower levels of growth hormone and insulin, which would make them grow more slowly.

Skin-to-skin contact reduces stress levels and endorphin levels of this kind of contact. It has been shown that the more the baby experiences of this kind of contact in the first six months of his life, the greater his or her mental development. The best kind of contact appears to be gentle but firm, and slow stroking. If the touch is too light it may irritate the child. And where you do the stroking also has its specific effect. If it is done on the back and on the legs the child will relax, but stroking the face, belly, or feet will stimulate him.

THE IMMUNE SYSTEM AND AGING

Hormones play a big role in the process of aging. The first time we suspected this was when we observed that elderly people who had strong family and neighborhood support systems appeared to be more able to fight off infections and recover from illness than those who were socially isolated.

We now believe that this is because people who are alone release more cortisol (the stress hormone) into their bodies, which impairs the immune system, raises blood pressure, and elevates heart rate. Widowed men, for example, may have a low white blood cell count and hence impaired immunity for fourteen months or more after their wives die. When older people are allowed to run their own lives and take care of everyday tasks they also seem to do much better. Because feelings of helplessness and uselessness are reduced, stress is reduced, and cortisol levels drop.

In contrast to increased cortisol levels, the elderly suffer from reduced levels of other hormones. There may be a drop in the level of hormones called thymosins that are produced by the thymus tissue and control the immune system. These substances were shown to boost the immune systems in a group of elderly people who could not fight off a case of influenza caused by a vaccine. They did this by making the bodies of these people produce larger numbers of antibodies to the disease. Because of this and other findings, researchers are now studying the effects of thymosins with a view to their possible use in the treatment of diseases such as AIDS, where the immune system has been severely impaired.

ADVANCES IN THE HORMONAL TREATMENT OF DISEASES
DIABETES

Diabetes is the most common hormonal disease, with about eleven million sufferers in the United States (see the Guide). These people either have too little insulin or their tissues become resistant to its action. The disease is usually treated with insulin, but daily or twice daily doses of the drug cannot keep a person's blood glucose levels as constant as they would be in someone not suffering from the disease. Sometimes the levels will rise too high and sometimes they will drop too low throughout the course of a day. In a normal person, the pancreas releases just enough insulin at all times to keep blood levels constant.

Because the complications of diabetes (heart disease, eye and leg problems, and so forth) are exacerbated by abnormal glucose levels, it would be best if we could find a type of treatment that would mimic the workings of a healthy pancreas. Well, new research is concentrating on getting other cells in the body to produce insulin in response to changing blood sugar levels. But let us backtrack here and explain some basics. All the cells in the body, no matter where they are found, have the same genes. That means that they all have the ability to produce insulin, in other words, they can all perform the jobs of any other cell. The reason why only the pancreatic cells do this particular job is because the other cells are stopped from doing it by what are called suppressor mechanisms in the body that are still not clearly understood. The new research is trying to find a way to turn off these suppressor mechanisms so that other tissues can respond to raised blood glucose levels by producing just the right amount of insulin.

HEART DISEASE

Whereas stress hormones increase blood pressure and heart rate, the heart itself produces hormones that reduce blood pressure by lowering blood volume. They do this by increasing the excretion of salt and water, which reduces the volume of the blood circulating in the vessels. They also relax the muscle in the walls of the arteries, which reduces the pressure within them. A new drug called auriculin, not yet released for general use, strongly resembles the structure of these hormones. It is hoped that this medication will become an effective treatment for both congestive heart failure and kidney malfunction (high blood pressure in the blood vessels of the kidneys damages them).

CANCER

Women who exercise vigorously in training for sporting events like the Olympics can experience delayed menstruation or irregular periods. They also seem to have a reduced susceptibility to breast, ovarian, and endometrial cancer.

There are two types of estrogen, estrone and estradiol, with the latter being much more active in the body than the former. Estrone, the less active form, seems to predominate in women who exercise vigorously, who have anorexia nervosa, and/or in those who have irregular periods. Recent studies have shown that women who exercise regularly are only half as likely to get these kinds of cancers. It would seem that the fewer the periods, the smaller the chance of developing these problems. Now this is not to say that overexercising or undereating is wise; far from it, as these situations can lead to other serious health problems. What this information could mean to experts in the future is that manipulation of these two estrogens might be used to treat or prevent these types of female cancers.

ENDOMETRIOSIS

Endometriosis affects one-third of all infertile women and is the third leading cause of infertility. As described in Chapter 6, it is marked by the movement of endometrial cells up the fallopian tubes and into the abdomen and other areas of the body. This can cause painful menstruation or abdominal pain throughout the second half of the menstrual cycle. It can also lead to scarring on the fallopian tubes, causing them to become blocked, and resulting in infertility. Recent studies suggest that endometriosis could be caused by a hormone called interleukin I, which is produced by the immune system as a reaction to the presence in the abdomen of cells from the uterus. Interleukin I increases the production of connective (scar) tissue which eventually blocks off the fallopian tubes. The hormone also suppresses bone growth and can lead to an abnormal loss of bone, resulting in osteoporosis.

At the present time, the treatments for endometriosis include a testosterone-like drug called danazol, gonadotropin releasing hormone (GRH), and surgery. Danazol causes weight gain, acne, deepening of the voice, and abnormal hair growth; GRH causes hot flashes and vaginal dryness; and surgery can be very painful. If a satisfactory way of suppressing interleukin I production could be found, it would be a superior form of treatment for the disease.

NEW METHODS OF BIRTH CONTROL

RU 486 is a new morning-after pill produced in France. It causes termination of a pregnancy by blocking the effects of progesterone (the hormone responsible for the thickening of the uterine wall to accommodate the growing fetus). It is effective in 80-85 percent of all cases if it is used in the first six weeks of pregnancy, but if used after nine or ten weeks after conception it only works in one-third of all women.

Prostaglandins made up the original morning-after pill. They were about 95 percent effective in bringing about a termination in the first three months of pregnancy by causing violent contractions of the uterus that ejected the embryo. But they also had drawbacks such as diarrhea, vomiting, and severe abdominal cramps. Because progesterone naturally blocks the ability of the prostaglandins to contract the uterus, high doses were needed to do the job.

RU 486 blocks the effects of progesterone and so by combining RU 486 with prostaglandins, much lower, safer doses of the latter substances can be given. RU 486 is given first, followed by an injection of prostaglandins two days later. This results in a miscarriage, which seems like a heavy period with only some cramps and slight nausea.

THE USES OF SYNTHETIC HORMONES

Hormones do not always have to be made in the body. At least these days they don't, and that fact is providing new and better ways of treating diseases. Hormones can now be made chemically or by genetic engineering, lowering their cost and increasing their availability and safety. Somatostatin is one such hormone. It controls the release of growth hormone and the secretion of intestinal hormones such as insulin and gastrin. When a benign tumor appears in the intestine and produces excess quantities of one or both of these intestinal hormones, serious problems can arise. For example, excess gastrin production can cause ulcers and excess insulin production can lead to hypoglycemia (see the Guide). Such tumors often grow very slowly and are inoperable. It is now becoming possible to prevent the problems caused by excess growth hormone or excesses of gastrointestinal hormones by giving synthetic somatostatin. These man-made hormones are more powerful than those normally produced by the body and successfully suppress the action of hormone-producing tumors.

Another hormone that has been successfully produced outside of the body is LRH (luteinizing releasing hormone). LRH is normally made by the hypothalamus and it stimulates the pituitary to produce LH (luteinizing hormone), which in turn stimulates estrogen or testosterone production. LRH is used to treat precocious puberty, prostate cancer, and benign tumors of the uterus. Synthetic forms of LRH are fifteen to twenty times stronger than natural LRH and so they can desensitize the pituitary to the actions of the natural hormone. These compounds can be used to stop estrogen production and help endometriosis; they can shrink fibrous uterine tumors by as much as 50 percent, which makes their dissection and removal possible and prevents the need for a hysterectomy. These LRH drugs can also be used to treat prostate cancer, as they stop the growth of the tumor and eliminate the need for removing the testicles.

The ability to produce synthetic hormones reduces the cost and dangers associated with extracting and using hormones from human tissues. For example, growth hormone used to be obtained from human pituitary glands taken from people's bodies after death. This was expensive and so it meant that very few children with growth hormone deficiency could be treated. And some of those who did receive natural hormone were infected with a slow-acting virus that eventually killed them. Today, genetic engineering has enabled us to produce enough safe, inexpensive growth hormone for everyone who needs it. And that is what the whole future of hormone research is about—treating and curing essential imbalances in the human body simply, cheaply, and completely.

PART TWO

A GUIDE
TO HORMONES
AND HORMONAL
PROBLEMS

HOW TO USE THIS GUIDE

This part of the book is set up as an easy-to-use reference guide to hormones and hormonal problems. The first section includes a list of the endocrine glands and the abbreviations for some of the more commonly discussed hormones. This is followed by tables alphabetically listing the hormones that are secreted by each gland, as well as each hormone's function in the body.

The second section of the Guide provides a listing of hormonal problems broken down into categories, such as "Sexual Development Abnormalities." You can use this as a cross-referencing tool: thus, if you are looking for a specific abnormality of sexual development, but are not sure of what the disorder is called, this listing will help you find the particular disorder you wish to learn about. The hormonal disorders are then presented alphabetically; each disorder is discussed in terms of its definition, incidence, diagnosis, signs and symptoms, and methods of treatment. In addition, a case history is included for each hormonal imbalance to provide you with as full a picture as possible of what can go wrong and what you can do about it.

THE ENDOCRINE SYSTEM: A REFERENCE LIST

Adrenals
Gastrointestional System
Gonads
Hypothalamus
Kidneys
Pancreas
Parathyroid
Pineal Gland
Pituitary
Prostaglandins
Thymus
Thyroid

ABBREVIATIONS FOR VARIOUS HORMONES

HORMONE	ABBREVIATION
Adrenocorticotropic Hormone	ACTH
Corticotropin Releasing Hormone	CRH
Follicle Stimulating Hormone	FSH
Gondaotropin Releasing Hormone	GnRH
Growth Hormone	GH
Growth Hormone Releasing Hormone	GRH
Lipotropins	LPH
Luteinizing Hormone	LH
Melanocyte Stimulating Hormone Inhibiting Factor	MIF
Melanocyte Stimulating Hormone	MSH
Parathyroid Hormone	PTH
Prolactin Release Inhibiting Hormone	PIH
Prolactin Releasing Factor	PRF
Renal Erythropoietic Factor	REF
Somatostatin	GHRIH
Thyroid Stimulating Hormone	TSH
Thyrotropin Releasing Hormone	TRH
Thyroxine	T4
Triiodothyronine	T3
Vasopressin	ADH

CHAPTER TEN

THE GLANDS AND THEIR HORMONES

ADRENALS

These are two glands, situated on top of the kidneys; each gland has two parts: the medulla and the cortex. They prepare the body for fight or flight, aid in metabolism.

HORMONE   **ACTION**

Adrenal Medulla:

Dopamine   Increases amount of blood pumped by the heart; increases amount of blood going to the kidneys.

Enkephalins and Somatostatin actions unknown, but one of the enkephalins (met-enkephalin) may be responsible for the addiction to nicotine.

Epinephrine increases heart rate, and the force of contraction of the heart. Dilates the coronary, muscle, kidney, and lung arterioles. Relaxes muscles in the lungs allowing freer breathing; relaxes muscles in the digestive system, slowing down the transit of food; relaxes the muscle in the wall of the bladder. Increases the secretion of hormones and digestive enzymes by the pancreas. Decreases blood glucose levels. Increases blood fat levels.

Norepinephrine increases sweating and thickness of saliva. Dilates the pupils. Constricts the coronary arteries; constricts the small arteries called arterioles in the skin, muscle, kidney, and digestive system. Constricts the small veins called venules throughout the body. Helps move food through the digestive system. By contracting the sphincter muscles in the anus, helps regulate bowel movements. Causes ejaculation in men. Decreases the secretion of hormones and digestive juices by the pancreas. Makes a person more alert, fearful, and anxious.

Adrenal Cortex:

Aldosterone	Helps maintain blood pressure by causing the kidneys to retain water. Helps maintain optimal sodium concentrations in the body.
Cortisol	Needed to excrete excess water from the body. Increases blood glucose levels. Causes breakdown of body protein. Decreases inflammation.

GASTROINTESTINAL SYSTEM

The entire digestive system—from the alimentary canal to the stomach and large and small intestines—secretes hormones that cause food to be broken down and allow the body to absorb required nutrients.

HORMONE	ACTION
Bombesin	Released in the small intestine and controls the release of gastrin and cholecystokinin. Helps control appetite.
Cholecystokinin	Stimulates the gall bladder, releases digestive juices from the pancreas, and helps control appetite. Secreted from the upper end of the small intestine.

Gastric Inhibitory Peptide	Inhibits the secretion of gastric acid. Secreted from the upper end of the small intestine.
Gastrin	Releases acid from the walls of the stomach. Secreted by the stomach and upper end of the small intestine.
Motilin	Secreted by cells from all parts of the intestine and causes accelerated movement of food along its length.
Neurotensin	Comes from the upper small intestine and inhibits the movement of the intestine. Slows down the movement of food along the length of the intestine.
Secretin	Releases bicarbonate and digestive juices from the pancreas.
Vasoactive Intestinal Peptide	Comes from all parts of the intestine, causes diarrhea and lowers blood pressure.

GONADS

These are the sex organs—the ovaries in women, the testes in men; they are responsible for reproduction and for sexual characteristics.

HORMONE	ACTION
In Women:	
Estrogen and Progesterone	Control the menstrual cycle and fertility; give a woman soft skin, breasts. Provide protection from heart disease. Prepare body for pregnancy; facilitate birth.
Relaxin	Aids in the birth process.

In Men:

Testosterone and related androgens	Responsible for growth of facial hair, deepening of voice, increasing muscular development. Control aggressiveness. Control sexual desire.

HYPOTHALAMUS

Located in the cerebral cortex of the brain, the hypothalamus is the regulator gland; it produces hormones that control the pituitary.

HORMONE	ACTION
Corticotropin Releasing Hormone (CRH)	Stimulates the release of corticotropin (ACTH) by the anterior pituitary.
Gonadotropin Releasing Hormone (also called Luteinizing Hormone Releasing Hormone— (GnRH, LHRH)	Causes the anterior pituitary to produce and release luteinizing hormone (LH) and follicle stimulating hormone (FSH).
Growth Hormone Releasing Hormone (GRH)	Stimulates the release of growth hormone by the anterior pituitary.
Melanocyte Stimulating Hormone Inhibiting Factor (MIF)	Inhibits the release of melanocyte stimulating hormone by the anterior pituitary.
Prolactin Release Inhibiting Hormone (PIH)	Inhibits the release of prolactin by the anterior pituitary.
Prolactin Releasing Factor (PRF)	Stimulates the release of prolactin by the anterior pituitary.

Somatostatin (Growth Hormone Release Inhibiting Hormone, or GHRIH)	Inhibits growth hormone release by a direct action on the anterior pituitary.
Thyrotropin Releasing Hormone (TRH)	Causes secretion of both thyroid stimulating hormone (TSH) and prolactin by the anterior pituitary.

Note: To understand how these hormonal actions affect our bodies, see the table on the pituitary hormones.

KIDNEYS

There are two kidneys. Besides excreting waste products of metabolism, they produce hormones that function to control blood pressure and blood manufacture.

HORMONE	ACTION
Renal erythropoietic factor (REF)	Controls the production of red blood cells.
Renin	Maintains normal blood pressure.

PANCREAS

Located behind the stomach, this gland regulates the body's glucose level.

HORMONE	ACTION
Glucagon	Raises blood glucose.
Insulin	Lowers blood glucose; necessary for absorption of glucose, without which, cells would die.

Pancreatic Polypeptide or   Roles not yet known.
Somatostatin

PARATHYROIDS

These four small glands on each side of the thyroid have a single purpose: to produce parathyroid hormone.

HORMONE	ACTION
Parathyroid hormone	Helps restore a low blood calcium level.

PINEAL GLAND

A small gland in the middle of the brain, the pineal produces the hormone responsible for skin and hair color; its other roles are not fully understood at this time, although it seems to function to inhibit the release of other hormones and may initiate puberty.

HORMONE	ACTION
Melatonin	Determines hair and skin color.

PITUITARY

Located below the hypothalamus, this gland consists of an anterior and a posterior lobe. It is the body's master gland.

HORMONE	ACTION
Anterior Pituitary:	
Adrenocorticotropic Hormone (ACTH)	Causes the adrenal cortex to produce cortisol. Involved in stress response.

Follicle Stimulating Hormone (FSH)	Stimulates estrogen production in the ovaries and sperm production in the testes.
Growth Hormone (GH)	Causes the liver to produce somatomedin which stimulates growth.
Lipotropins (LPH)	May relieve pain.
Luteinizing Hormone (LH)	Induces ovulation, stimulates estrogen and progesterone production from the ovaries and testosterone production from the testes.
Melanocyte Stimulating Hormone (MSH)	Stimulates the production of pigment in the skin.
Prolactin	Stimulates the breasts to grow and produce milk. Causes manufacture of body muscle.
Thyroid Stimulating Hormone	Stimulates the production and release (TSH) of thyroid hormones.
Posterior Pituitary:	
Oxytocin	Acts on the breasts to eject milk and causes the contractions of the uterus during birth.
Vasopressin (also called Antidiuretic Hormone, or ADH)	Acts on the kidneys to decrease urine production.

PROSTAGLANDINS

These are not glands, but are hormones themselves, which are produced from linoleic acid, a type of fat found in our diet. Prostaglandins have been found in semen, in the kidneys, uterus, blood cells, joints, and other tissues.

HORMONE	ACTION
Prostaglandin	Control many reactions. Responsible for labor, menstruation, clotting, and immunity.

THYMUS

This gland, located behind the breastbone, has a vital—if not the most important—role in the body's immune system.

HORMONE	ACTION
Thymosin	Activates lymphocytes, enabling them to destroy microorganisms that cause disease—in other words, activates the immune system.

THYROID

This butterfly-shaped gland is essential to metabolism and plays a major role in growth.

HORMONE	ACTION
Calcitonin	Keeps blood calcium levels from increasing abnormally.
Thyroxine (T4) and Triiodothyronine (T3)	Regulate the metabolism; speed up the activity of all body organs except the brain, testes, spleen, and anterior pituitary.

CHAPTER ELEVEN

KNOWING THE FACTS
BOUT HORMONAL DISEASES

The whole purpose of this book is for you to understand the intricate workings of your hormonal system better and to see how vital this system is to your mental and physical health. Even minor hormonal imbalances can lead to major symptoms and serious health problems. Having said that, you should also know something else: Many hormonal problems have very few symptoms, or relatively minor ones. Therefore, if something does change in your appearance or your body, you should not just dismiss it but instead see your doctor, just to make sure the cause of this "slight" problem is not a hormonal one.

Hormonal disorders are one of those things most often missed by the layperson. A little more hair than usual falls out, or there is a slight pain in the wrist, or perhaps the nose or jaw suddenly seems a bit more prominent. Maybe your weight is going up or down when your diet is remaining the same. Or perhaps you find yourself urinating more than usual and seized by an uncontrollable thirst. These are all symptoms of hormonal disorders and some of them, if left untreated, can result in severe complications.

Of course, hair loss may also be caused by simple stress, weight gain by unconscious overeating, and pain in the wrists by awkward movements during the playing of certain sports. But you will not know whether or not the problem is a serious one unless you see your physician. If your doctor cannot readily find the cause and suspects a hormonal imbalance, he or she can refer you to an endocrinologist, who may then take a series of sophisticated and accurate tests.

All hormonal problems can be treated in some way, and most if not all of the symptoms can disappear after treatment. The trick is not to leave the problem alone for too long and dismiss the symptoms as part of aging, or daily stress, or just a case of hypochondria.

One final note on this section: so that you can see in actual practice how hormonal problems affect your life and how they can be diagnosed and treated, each of the sections concerning a specific ailment contains a case history. The names of these patients have been changed, but the circumstances surrounding their diseases and subsequent medical care are authentic.

HORMONAL PROBLEMS: A REFERENCE LIST

Adrenal Gland Disorders
  Adrenocorticol Insufficiency (Addison's Disease)
  Cushing's Syndrome
  Phaeochromocytoma
  Primary Aldosteronism (Conn's Syndrome)

Bone Disorders
  Osteoporosis
  Rickets and Osteomalacia

Diabetes Mellitus

Parathyroid Disorders
  Hyperparpthyroidism
  Hypoparathyroidism

Pituitary Disorders
  Acromegaly or Gigantism (Excess Growth Hormone)
  Diabetes Insipidus
  Hypopituitarism

Sexual Development Abnormalities
  Delayed Puberty
  Precocious Puberty

Sexual Function Abnormalities
  Amenorrhea (Failure to Menstruate)
  Gynecomastia
  Hirsutism
  Impotence
  Infertility

Thyroid Disorders
  Hypothyroidism
  Hyperthyroidism
  Thyroid Nodules (including Thyroid Cancer)

THE DISORDERS

ACROMEGALY OR GIGANTISM (EXCESS GROWTH HORMONE)

DEFINITION

An excess of growth hormone leads to a disorder called gigantism in children and acromegaly in adults. In this condition there is an enlargement of most organs of the body.

HOW COMMON IS IT?

This disorder affects only one person in 40,000.

CAUSES

Growth hormone works by stimulating the liver to produce growth-promoting hormones called somatomedins. Those who suffer from acromegaly or gigantism have an oversecretion of growth hormone resulting in an excess of somatomedins. This excessive secretion is usually the result of a benign tumor in the pituitary.

CASE HISTORY

Michael Duggan, 43, a bank teller, was married and had a seven-year-old daughter. He went to see his doctor, complaining that for the last three months he had been sweating abnormally and his fingers were extremely stiff and painful. While he had not been eating any more than usual he had gained six pounds over the last six weeks. He was also suffering from headaches, and over the past six months he had gradually lost interest in sex.

Although the doctor had treated Michael since he was a child, he hadn't seen him in many years. He immediately noticed that Michael's jaw was protruding and his facial features were coarser, with thicker lips and a more prominent nose and ears. His blood pressure and heart rate were both above normal, and his vision was slightly impaired.

The doctor suspected acromegaly. A blood test for growth hormone revealed abnormally high levels which failed to drop after Michael drank a glucose solution. A CAT scan showed the presence of a tumor on his pituitary. Michael was referred to a neurosurgeon who removed the benign growth. Michael then went into remission. His facial features returned to normal but he was left with enlarged hands.

SIGNS AND SYMPTOMS

Gigantism or excessively tall stature occurs if the disease develops before a person's bones have fully formed in length. Heights may reach over eight feet. If the disease appears after growth has been completed (then called acromegaly), the bones widen instead. Broadening of the hands and feet leads to increases in ring size, glove size, and shoe size over the years. This is very obvious when the hand of such a person is shaken in greeting: you get the feeling of losing your own hand in a mass of dough because of the other's size and fleshiness. For a person with this disease, joint pain, numbness, and tingling in the hands are also common. Facial features are coarse with furrowed brows, prominent lines joining the outside of the nose to the corners of the mouth, and a wide, projecting nose. The lower jaw elongates and projects outward. Wide spaces develop between the teeth. The person sweats heavily and the skin becomes very greasy. The tongue, lips, and ears enlarge. Overgrowth of the tissue causes pain in the wrist due to pressure on the nerves. The vocal cords also thicken, leading to a deepening of the voice. The person may also suffer from deep-seated headaches, loss of sex drive, and visual problems.

Internal abnormalities are also found. The heart and liver enlarge and high blood pressure frequently occurs. While muscle tissue also grows, acromegalic persons are usually physically weak. Osteoporosis (brittle bones) afflicts many of these people. A goiter (enlarged thyroid) is often present. About one-quarter of acromegalic patients have diabetes mellitus; another 20 percent show signs of developing it. This, combined with the cardiovascular problems suffered by these people, accounts for their reduced life expectancy.

All of these changes occur very slowly in an acromegalic person and may progress for years before the subtle differences can be noticed by using "before and after" snapshots of the person. All children with gigantism are subject to the same symptoms as the adults.

METHODS OF DIAGNOSIS

Acromegaly is diagnosed by observing the changes in appearance and body structure described above and confirming the diagnosis by measuring the blood levels of growth hormone after an overnight fast and after giving the patient a solution of glucose to drink. A rise in blood glucose normally suppresses the growth hormone secretion but in acromegaly this does not happen—and hormone levels may even rise.

TREATMENT

Acromegaly is treated with surgery or radiation to remove or destroy the tumor that is secreting growth hormone. Surgery is the best form of treatment if the tumor is small. (The smaller the tumor, the greater the chance of successful remission.) External irradiation can be successful although it can take several years. The patients usually come through this treatment quite well with just temporary hair loss and nausea. Alternatively, a radioactive compound can be implanted into the pituitary. The main problem here is the possibility of causing hypopituitarism, which may require hormone replacement therapy.

About 20 percent of acromegalics can be successfully treated with a drug called bromocriptine. As soon as the drug is stopped, however, growth hormone levels usually rise again, and so this form of treatment is usually combined with one of the other methods.

When the person has been successfully treated, the symptoms (coarsened appearance, sweating, numbness of hand, joint pains, diabetes) are usually relieved but the enlargement of the hands and feet often remain. Gigantism is generally treated in the same way as acromegaly.

ADDISON'S DISEASE
(SEE ADRENOCORTICOL INSUFFICIENCY)
ADRENOCORTICOL INSUFFICIENCY
(ADDISON'S DISEASE)

DEFINITION

In this disorder, the adrenal glands cannot produce normal amounts of cortisol.

HOW COMMON IS IT?

One in 10,000 people have this disorder.

CAUSES

Ninety percent of all Addison's patients have an autoimmune disease called autoimmune adrenalitis, in which their own immune systems destroy the cells of the adrenal cortex. This disease is often found in the same people who have Hashimoto's disease (see Hypothyroidism in the Guide) and/or anemia, and less frequently in people who have diabetes mellitus (also discussed in the Guide), ovarian failure, and hyperparathyroidism (also discussed in the Guide).

When the disease was first discovered in 1881, destruction of the adrenal glands due to tuberculosis was the main cause and is still a major culprit in countries where tuberculosis is common. Other diseases, such as fungal infections and cancer, can also have the same effect.

CASE HISTORY

Stanley Rogers, a thirty-six-year-old accountant, noticed over the last two months that he seemed to be getting more and more tired and actually felt physically weak at times. When he could no longer work for more than a few hours without needing rest, he went to see his doctor. The doctor immediately saw that Stan was extremely thin. His blood pressure readings were below normal and when asked to stand he admitted that he felt a little giddy, as though he'd had a few too many drinks. Though he looked very pale, there were some areas of dark discoloration on the inside of his lips and on the roof of his mouth.

The doctor did a series of blood tests on Stan and found that he had low blood sodium, calcium, and chloride levels, and high blood potassium, urea, and cortisol levels. The blood cortisol measurement was repeated after Stan was put through a stress test, and this showed that the levels did not rise the way they should have.

Suspecting Addison's disease, the doctor next did a synacthen test which confirmed his suspicions. An additional blood test showed antibodies against adrenal tissue. Stan was finally diagnosed with autoimmune adrenalitis. He was immediately placed on hydrocortisone to be taken in the morning and at night, and his urine cortisol levels were measured from time to time to make sure the dosage was correct. Stan soon felt much better and more than able to handle the pressures of the coming tax season.

SIGNS AND SYMPTOMS
- Extreme weakness and fatigue
- Gastrointestinal disturbances, including lack of appetite, nausea, and even vomiting, leading to weight loss
- Vague stomach ache
- A craving for salt (20 percent of cases)
- Dizziness upon standing, even fainting
- Skin color is extremely pale but becomes darker (more pigment) wherever it is subject to friction at skin creases on the knuckles, elbows, and knees; exposed to the sun; exposed to pressure from belts and straps; has any old scars; and at the nipples and surrounding areas, the scrotum, the buttocks, inside the lips, and on the roof of the mouth
- Women may tend to lose hair from under their arms and the pubic region.

Stress can cause the symptoms of this disease to become life-threatening. For more on this, see the Treatment section.

METHODS OF DIAGNOSIS
Any person with an unexplained weight loss should be suspected of possibly having Addison's disease. It becomes even more likely when the person has the signs and symptoms mentioned above and has low blood pressure that gets worse upon standing up from a sitting or lying position.

When a person has these symptoms, the doctor will measure blood cortisol levels when he or she is under stress. The level in a normal person will rise significantly under such circumstances, but this will not happen in anyone with this disorder. The presence of low blood sodium, calcium, and chloride levels and high blood potassium and urea levels would tend to confirm the diagnosis. But to be absolutely sure, the doctor would also do a synacthen (commercially produced ACTH) test in which the person is given an intramuscular injection of the substance and then blood cortisol levels are measured at the time of the injection and at one, four, eight, and twenty-four hours afterwards. If the person has this disease the adrenal glands will be unable to respond normally to the ACTH, which is by making large amounts of cortisol.

Once the diagnosis is made, the doctor must determine the cause. If the patient is female and has a history of autoimmune diseases in her family, then the chances are that she has autoimmune adrenalitis. She may even have antibodies in her blood to adrenal tissue, although this is not always the case. If there is no family history of autoimmune diseases, then an x-ray may reveal tuberculosis or cancer.

TREATMENT

In a normal person, the levels of blood cortisol are highest in the morning and lowest at night. When patients are treated for Addison's disease they are given cortisol in the form of hydrocortisone or cortisone acetate and the doctor tries to mimic the body's normal response by giving twice as much in the morning as at night. He will then periodically monitor the cortisol level in the urine to make sure the dosage is not too high, which could cause Cushing's syndrome (see later section of the Guide). People with Addison's disease also commonly need aldosterone replacement therapy as well. This is given once a day or every other day in the form of fludrocortisone, as needed. If too much of this is given the person will develop high blood pressure and water retention causing swelling in various parts of the body such as the ankles, breasts, and around the eyes.

Stress can exacerbate the symptoms of adrenocortical insufficiency and make them life-threatening. Such stress might come in the form of a serious infection, a major operation, or the birth of a child. When subjected to these conditions, the person who already has the disease may vomit uncontrollably, become severely dehydrated, and lose so much fluid from the body that the blood pressure drops to critically low levels. This will mean that the vital organs cannot be supplied with enough blood and will result in a coma. Such a situation is a true medical emergency, since the person in the coma may die within twenty-four hours. The stricken patient is immediately given hydrocortisone intravenously along with an intravenous solution of sodium chloride.

For those in treatment, this dangerous scenario can be avoided by anticipating stressful situations and increasing the dosage of hormone replacement therapy (as per instructions by the physician) both prior to and during the period of stress. Because of this problem, all people on cortisol therapy either carry a card or wear a necklace at all times that indicates they are on this medication.

AMENORRHEA
(FAILURE TO MENSTRUATE)

DEFINITION

There are two different types of amenorrhea, which is the medical term used to describe a woman's failure to menstruate. Primary amenorrhea is the failure to menstruate by the age of sixteen and is covered more extensively in the Guide section, "Delayed Puberty." Secondary amenorrhea is the absence of menstrual periods for more than three months in a woman who has previously menstruated normally.

HOW COMMON IS IT?

Almost every woman who has lived to sixty years of age has experienced amenorrhea at some point in her life. Many women have long lapses between periods during the first year or two after puberty, or when they begin to go into menopause. Others only experience amenorrhea when they become pregnant, where it is part of the normal reproductive changes occurring at this time. Apart from the extremes of puberty and menopause, however, there are a variety of conditions that can cause amenorrhea. Excessive weight loss is responsible for 20 percent of the cases of secondary amenorrhea, excess prolactin release can account for another 20 percent, and 1 to 2 percent of all women have this problem when they first stop using oral contraceptives.

CAUSES

Secondary amenorrhea in premenopausal women is most often caused by pregnancy. If this is not the case, then a defect in gonadotropin secretion caused by obesity, anorexia (a woman of 5'5" in height will not menstruate if her weight falls below 108 pounds—see Table 4 in Chapter 4), stress, chronic illness affecting the pituitary's response to GnRH, or vigorous exercise are all possible culprits. Vigorous training and exercise can cause amenorrhea because of a loss of body fat. To maintain normal periods, a woman needs to have a lean to fat body weight of about 2.5 to 1, whereas body builders, who can easily suffer from amenorrhea, often have a ratio of 4 to 1. Another common cause is an excessive production of prolactin, usually produced because of a tumor on the pituitary. Secondary amenorrhea can also be the result of a number of conditions affecting one of more of the endocrine glands, including tumors on the hypothalamus or ovaries; enlarged cystic ovaries; ovarian failure due to exposure to chemotherapy, x-ray therapy, surgical removal, or an autoimmune disease (where the woman produces antibodies that destroy her own ovaries); tuberculosis in the lining of the uterus, or fibrous tissue invading this lining; thyroid disease; adrenal disease; breastfeeding; use of oral contraceptives; use of the phenothiazine family of antipsychotic drugs; heavy use of alcohol or tobacco; or nutritional deficiencies.

CASE HISTORY
    Miranda is twenty-three years old and a recent college graduate. Before going out on her first set of job interviews, she decided that to look her very best, she had to lose some weight. She began an intensive course of aerobic exercise for three hours each day, at the same time eating no more than a meager diet of cake, french fries, and the occasional dinner out with her boyfriend. Her periods soon became irregular, but she ignored the problem, figuring it would eventually straighten itself out.
    She was thrilled but at the same time very nervous when she got her first job at a major television company. Shortly after she started working there, her periods stopped altogether. At first she thought she was pregnant, but the tests came up negative. After four months of amenorrhea, she got the name of an endocrinologist from a co-worker and went to see him.
    The doctor gave her a full physical examination and while weighing her saw that she had lost 15 percent of her ideal body weight. He explained to her that although she was not alarmingly thin, her loss of body fat was interfering with her ability to menstruate because it upset the normal functioning of her hypothalamus in ways that are not yet understood. This problem, added to the stress of her new job, was probably causing the amenorrhea.
    Miranda started to eat normally and reduced her exercise program

from excessive to moderate. She also began to feel more comfortable in her job. After a weight gain of only five pounds, she started to menstruate normally again.

SIGNS AND SYMPTOMS
A chief sign is a failure to menstruate for at least three months. There may also be signs of the underlying condition causing the problem, such as secretion of milk from the breasts if there is excess prolactin release, or overuse of a phenothiazine tranquilizer; or dryness of the vagina and pain during intercourse in women with low estrogen levels. You should also know that if low levels of estrogen are not treated for a long period of time there is an increased risk of getting osteoporosis (brittle bones).

METHODS OF DIAGNOSIS
If there is no obvious reason for secondary amenorrhea (pregnancy, severe weight loss, obesity, vigorous exercise, chronic illness, or stress), the physician will carry out a number of tests. Initially, progesterone will be given to the patient. If menstrual bleeding then occurs, it means that the pituitary, hypothalamus, and ovaries are all functioning normally, but the lining of the uterus has shrunken (often due to prolonged use of oral contraceptive agents containing progesterone).

If bleeding does not occur, it means that either the pituitary, hypothalamus, or ovaries are not functioning properly. If this is the case the blood is then measured for LH, FSH, estrogen, and testosterone levels. Low FSH, LH, and estrogen levels point to a pituitary or hypothalamic problem that may need to be examined further with such tests as a CAT scan to rule out tumors. Low or normal levels of FSH with elevated LH, testosterone, or other androgens usually means a cystic ovary. Elevated testosterone levels alone suggest ovarian tumors or adrenal disease.

If thyroid disease is suspected, T3, T4, and TSH levels will also be checked.

TREATMENT
Patients with tumors are surgically treated. Antithyroid drugs or radioactive iodine are given to patients with hyperthyroidism; cortisol is given to patients with adrenal insufficiency; estrogens are given to those with ovarian failure; and gonadotropins are given to women with

gonadotropin deficiency. Obese patients are encouraged to lose weight and underweight patients to gain some. Pain during intercourse can be treated with an estrogen-based cream (such as Estrace, Ogen). Women with high prolactin levels are given a dopamine-like medication (bromocriptine, brand name: Parlodel) that prevents prolactin release. (Dopamine is a chemical that acts as a neurotransmitter, or messenger, in the central nervous system.)

After stopping the use of oral contraceptive agents, normal periods should resume in a matter of a few months. If they do not, further medical investigation may be required.

CUSHING'S SYNDROME

DEFINITION
The adrenal gland is divided into two parts, called the cortex and the medulla. The medulla is the core of the gland and is surrounded by the cortex, which produces the adrenocortical hormones—cortisol, the androgens, estrogens, and aldosterone. Oversecretion of these hormones leads to a disease called Cushing's syndrome.

HOW COMMON IS IT?
One in 20,000 people have this disease. It is most common in women (ten times more common than in men) and especially in young and middle-aged women (from twenty to forty years of age). It is rarely found in children or the elderly.

CAUSES
Cushing's syndrome can have many different causes. The most common one is overdosage with corticosteroids, taken for a variety of reasons such as arthritis, Crohn's disease, and body building. Apart from this, the major cause is the excess production of ACTH by a benign tumor (an adenoma) in the pituitary gland. Other reasons for the development of the disease include: a benign or malignant (more common in children) tumor in the adrenal cortex that produces excess cortisol; or the production of ACTH by a cancerous tumor in another part of the body outside of the pituitary gland (most commonly in the lung, but it can also be in the thymus, pancreas, ovaries, or thyroid), which is called an ectopic tumor.

CASE HISTORY

Audrey Jenkins, a thirty-five-year-old salesperson, went to see her doctor complaining of frequent headaches, depression, irregular menstrual periods, pains in her arms and legs, frequent urination, and the development of a protruding stomach. Audrey was very upset with the way her appearance had recently changed; not only had she become obese, but her body had taken on a peculiar shape unlike other heavy women she observed in her health club.

The doctor examined Audrey and found that she had abnormally high blood pressure, thin and dry skin, and bruises over her legs. Her arms and legs were also very thin. A blood screening test showed high glucose levels and low potassium levels. Urine analyses taken on three separate days showed a consistently high level of cortisol.

Audrey's doctor suspected Cushing's syndrome, and since she was not taking any kind of medication that could cause the disorder, he gave her an overnight dexamethasone test. This showed an abnormally high level of blood cortisol. He followed it up by giving Audrey two milligrams of dexamethasone four times a day for two days and found that her blood cortisol levels went down to normal, indicating that she had a pituitary tumor. A CAT scan confirmed this. Audrey was operated on for the removal of the tumor and by six months later she had lost the extra weight she'd gained and was back to normal again.

SIGNS AND SYMPTOMS

People with Cushing's syndrome have a characteristic appearance:
- Large stomach;
- Rounded back due to the deposition of fat (known as a buffalo's hump);
- Flushed, round, and fat moon face;
- Fat neck; and
- Abnormally thin arms and legs due to muscle wasting.

The person is said to resemble a "lemon on toothpicks," a distribution of weight that is very different from regular obesity where the person is fat all over the body. Other symptoms include:
- Thin and dry skin;
- Bruising easily;
- Wide purple bands over the stomach, back, and thighs;
- Discoloration of the skin;

- Hairiness;
- Puffy eyelids;
- Backache due to collapse of the back bone, and osteoporosis (see later section)
- Mood swings, depression, and even psychotic episodes;
- Diabetes mellitus (see later section of the Guide) for 60% of patients and high blood pressure;
- Acne and hirsutism (see later Guide section) in women, due to the excess production of androgens by the adrenal cortex, which also causes loss of the menstrual periods or irregular and scanty periods;
- Excess estrogen in men, which may cause impotence; and
- Growth retardation and obesity (the main signs in children).

The disease progresses insidiously and if left untreated or poorly controlled can lead to death within five years due to such things as strokes, heart attacks, infections, or complications from diabetes mellitus.

METHODS OF DIAGNOSIS

If a person is found to have the signs and symptoms just described, a screening blood test may show low potassium levels, excess red blood cells, and abnormally alkaline blood. Tests of the urine done on three different occasions may reveal consistently raised cortisol levels. In order to confirm the presence of Cushing's syndrome, an overnight dexamethasone suppression test is done. Dexamethasone is a potent, cortisol-like substance which in a normal person will inhibit the secretion of CRF by the hypothalamus and ACTH by the pituitary. Hence, there will be less ACTH available to stimulate the adrenal glands to produce their hormones and cortisol levels will go down. However, when a person has a tumor producing ACTH in his pituitary, this is not inhibited by the dexamethasone and blood cortisol levels will remain high. In this test, the dexamethasone is given at bedtime and blood cortisol levels are measured the next morning.

A more complicated dexamethasone test may be done to distinguish between the different causes of Cushing's syndrome. Whereas it takes 0.5 milligrams of dexamethasone taken four times a day for forty-eight hours to suppress cortisol production in normal people, it takes 2 milligrams taken four times a day for forty-eight hours to suppress cortisol production caused by excess ACTH produced by a pituitary tumor. However, even this amount will not prevent cortisol production caused by an adrenal or ectopic tumor that secretes ACTH.

Another way of differentiating between causes of the disease is to take a measurement of ACTH in the blood in the morning and at midnight. Both levels will be high if a pituitary adenoma or ectopic tumor is responsible for the disorder, and low if there is an adrenal tumor. Someone with an adrenal tumor will also tend to grow a lot of hair and women will develop more masculine traits such as a beard and a low-pitched voice. People who have a lung tumor will often lose weight rather than gain it and become extremely skinny, and their blood potassium levels will be very low.

Other important diagnostic tests include chest x-rays to look for lung tumors, and x-rays of the kidney area for adrenal tumors. When an adrenal tumor is present, the underlying kidney may be pushed down or the tumor may even grow into the kidney.

TREATMENT

If the disease has been caused by a pituitary adenoma, the removal of this benign tumor is the treatment of choice in adults. Cyproheptadine, a drug that inhibits CRF production by the hypothalamus (and in turn inhibits ACTH release by the pituitary), has occasionally gotten rid of the symptoms. In children, irradiation of the pituitary is the preferred treatment.

If the disease is caused by an adrenal tumor, the treatment is the surgical removal of the affected gland.

If the culprit is ectopic ACTH production, removal of the tumor producing the excess ACTH is often not possible because it may be very small at first and difficult to find, and so drugs that inhibit the production of cortisol (such as aminoglutethimide and metyraprone) are used.

DELAYED PUBERTY

DEFINITION

Most girls and boys begin to show signs of puberty by the ages of thirteen and thirteen and a half, respectively. Therefore, sexual development taking place after age fourteen in girls and fifteen in boys is called delayed puberty.

HOW COMMON IS IT?

Two percent of all girls do not start developing breasts by thirteen years of age and two percent of boys fail to experience enlargement of the testicles by thirteen and a half. Most of these children do enter puberty within one or two years, although it is not unusual for sexual development to be delayed until the age of eighteen. When children without an underlying disorder do eventually enter puberty, they grow to a normal height, mature normally, and show no hormonal abnormalities. This type of late puberty is called constitutional growth delay. It is six times more common in boys than in girls. It also often runs in families, which would tend to show that some genetic factor must be delaying the secretion of gonadotropins.

Children who fall outside this category have a more serious condition and will most likely require medical treatment to induce puberty.

CAUSES

As just mentioned, genetic factors could play a role in the development of constitutional growth delay. Nonconstitutional cases are either caused by a reduced production of GnRH or by a failure on the part of the gonads to produce sex hormones. The former problem is often caused by chronic diseases which can affect the hypothalamus such as asthma, celiac disease, tuberculosis, Crohn's disease, or thalassemia. Eating disorders that involve starvation (such as anorexia nervosa), intensive physical training (as seen in ballet dancers or marathon runners), or emotional stress can also have the same effect. Rarer causes are congenital defects in the development of the hypothalamus (where delayed puberty is often accompanied by a lack of the sense of smell, a harelip, or cleft palate), diseases of the pituitary, underdeveloped sex organs, overdeveloped adrenals, an underactive thyroid, diabetes, or chromosomal abnormalities.

CASE HISTORY

For Fred, his sixteenth birthday was just another sad, lonely day spent with his parents. He had no girlfriends or even friends, because the kids at school thought he was "weird." Although he was not unusually tall, his arms and legs were noticeably out of proportion with his body. The other boys on his basketball team teased him in the locker room about his tiny penis and testes and his lack of body hair. His voice was high and effeminate, and although he knew he wasn't sexually interested in men, he wasn't very attracted to girls, either. After he turned sixteen, his parents brought him to the doctor because they, too, were growing more and more concerned about his lack of normal development. During medical questioning, Fred revealed something he had never even told his parents. "I can't smell anything," he said to the doctor, "but I figured that was just some little thing that made me different." The doctor thought otherwise and suspected an abnormality of the hypothalamus.

Fred's blood tests showed that he had low levels of gonadotropins and testosterone. He was given GnRH and finally began to develop normally. Because his condition was caught early, he did not become abnormally tall, although his arms and legs remained a little too long for the rest of his body.

SIGNS AND SYMPTOMS

In girls: Failure to develop breasts, lack of menstruation, absence of pubic and body hair.

In boys: Testes remain small, no deepening of the voice, absence of pubic and body hair.

If the problem is nonconstitutional, added symptoms appear. Because of the lack of androgens, boys who are not treated early enough will not grow correctly. The long bones in the arms and legs will grow for an abnormally long period and as a result, these children will be tall, but with limbs that are out of proportion with their bodies. In addition to having very long arms and legs, the boy will lay down fat on his hips and thighs—traits more characteristic of women. (This physical structure, by the way, appeared in eunuchs.) However, despite the lack of androgens, this enlarged skeleton will not develop in boys who have abnormally low levels of growth hormone or a genetic defect that predisposes them to a short stature. (Girls do not develop the enlarged skeleton.) Delayed puberty caused by genetic defects usually results in other physical abnormalities such as breast development in boys, and webbing of the neck, widely spaced nipples, and defects in the cardiovascular system in girls.

METHODS OF DIAGNOSIS

All children with delayed puberty should be checked for chronic diseases such as asthma that might explain their problems.

If puberty is late and the boy is not growing very well but the penis and testes are normal and the boy is healthy, it is most likely that he is a late bloomer with constitutional growth delay. In these cases, the physician will simply observe the child over the next six months before taking any tests. If the testes grow significantly during this time no treatment or tests are needed, except to watch the child closely and make sure normal sexual development continues. But if there is no sign of sexual growth during this time period, further tests may be done. Similarly, boys with accompanying physical abnormalities and girls with delayed puberty (with or without physical problems) will be given a variety of tests.

Blood samples will be taken to measure sex hormone, gonadotropin, thyroid hormone, and cortisol levels. When a disorder mainly affects the testes or ovaries, testosterone or estrogen levels will be low and LH and FSH levels will be elevated. This can be confirmed by testing the ability of the gonads to respond to gonadotropins. Injected FSH should cause ovulation in a girl which can be seen by an ultrasound imaging test. Testosterone measurements are made in boys before and after being given gonadotropin into the muscle (for three doses on alternate days). The testosterone levels should rise to the adult range if the testes are normal.

If pituitary disease is the culprit, LH and FSH levels will be low and any GnRH administered by the physician will not elevate them to any significant degree. Children with hypothalamic disease causing a lack of GnRH secretion will receive injections of GnRH for three days. This should stimulate a healthy pituitary to produce gonadotropins and so LH and FSH levels will rise. If hypothalamic or pituitary disease is suspected, a CAT scan will be done to look for tumors or structural defects.

When physical abnormalities are present in the child, a chromosomal analysis will be carried out to find any genetic defects.

An abnormal thyroid hormone or cortisol level would suggest thyroid or adrenal disease (see corresponding section of the Guide).

TREATMENT

Boys: If puberty does not occur, whatever the reason, it must be induced. This should be done somewhere between the ages of sixteen and eighteen, since the induction of puberty stops growth and may reduce adult height if done too early. If the testes grow and produce testosterone when the boy is given gonadotropins (in the form of HCG or human chorionic gonadotropin, extracted from a human placenta where it is produced to stimulate fetal growth), and the hypothalamus and pituitary seem normal, then puberty is induced by intramuscular injections of HCG twice weekly for six weeks. If this treatment fails, or if there is a testicular, pituitary, or hypothalamic problem, then puberty is induced gradually by first administering small and then larger oral doses of testosterone.

Girls: If all hormonal tests show normal levels, there is no hard and fast rule as to when puberty should be induced with doses of estrogen. If the girl is short, there is some risk that giving the treatment too early will further stunt her growth. However, because of psychological pressures, treatment will usually begin between the ages of fifteen and sixteen. However, if the delayed puberty is not constitutional and the child is of normal height, treatment may begin earlier.

To induce puberty, a very small oral dose of estrogen (such as five micrograms of ethinyl estradiol) is given and gradually increased over a twelve-month period in order to mimic the changes occurring in normal pubescence. The medication is then switched to a cyclical estrogen/progesterone mixture to induce menstruation. At this point, estrogen is given for fifteen days, and estrogen with progesterone is given on days fifteen to twenty-four. If, at the end of this treatment, the girl still does not menstruate, the hormones are given again, until menstruation occurs. Once the girl starts to develop normally, the dose is gradually reduced to the lowest amount needed to maintain regular monthly bleeding.

DIABETES INSIPIDUS

DEFINITION
This rare disease, not to be confused with diabetes mellitus (see the next section), is marked by an inability to conserve water, and so maintain the body's normal level of water.

HOW COMMON IS IT?
Although there are no statistics on how many people get this disease, it is known to be quite uncommon.

CAUSES
Diabetes insipidus can be caused by a deficiency of ADH (antidiuretic hormone, also called vasopressin). This hormone, produced by the posterior lobe of the pituitary, acts on the kidneys to make them conserve water. A deficiency of ADH may be inherited, or caused by a poor blood supply to the pituitary, an infection, damage caused by

accident or surgery, or a tumor. It can also happen because the kidney becomes less sensitive to the actions of ADH, and in this case it can also be inherited or arise as a result of the use of drugs such as lithium or demeclocycline.

CASE HISTORY

Bruce Spencer, a thirty-year-old high school teacher, was involved in a serious car accident, where he hit his head on the wheel and was knocked unconscious. Directly following that injury, he started to urinate at least eight times a day and had to wake up two or three times during the night to go to the bathroom. He was also developing an insatiable thirst. He told his doctor about these symptoms during one of his postaccident checkups. While the doctor found him to be generally healthy with a normal blood pressure and pulse, he went ahead and ordered a battery of tests, suspecting that something had happened because of Bruce's car accident. Blood tests ruled out diabetes mellitus, hypokalemia, hypercalcemia, and kidney disease, and so the doctor sent Bruce to the hospital for an eight-hour fluid deprivation test. The results of this test indicated that he had diabetes insipidus. A CAT scan then revealed that Bruce's head injury had damaged his pituitary gland. He was treated by being given DDAVP, the synthetic analog of ADH (a chemical made in a laboratory which has the same actions as ADH) which he sniffed up his nose. Bruce stopped urinating constantly and lost his insatiable thirst.

SIGNS AND SYMPTOMS

A huge amount of urine is excreted, causing a severe thirst during both night and day and leading to excessive drinking. The person becomes dehydrated unless the amount of fluid he consumes can match the amount he loses. Dryness of the mouth and skin, constipation (because there is too little water in the body to soften the stool), weakness, and fatigue are other symptoms.

METHODS OF DIAGNOSIS

The main goal of the tests is to differentiate between diabetes insipidus and other causes of excessive urination and thirst (diabetes mellitus, hypercalcemia or high blood calcium levels, hypokalemia or low blood potassium levels, kidney disease, and a psychiatric disorder known as compulsive water drinking). Urine testing and blood glucose measurements will eliminate diabetes mellitus. Hypokalemia, which can be caused by diarrhea, vomiting, or the use of diuretics, can be detected by a simple blood test. Hypercalcemia found in the blood leads to a search for its causes, which can include hyperparathyroidism (see later section of the Guide), cancer, or the excess consumption of vitamin D. If blood urea levels are raised, then a kidney problem will be suspected and investigated further.

If none of these other tests show anything abnormal, then the field is narrowed down to either compulsive water drinking or diabetes insipidus. In the former instance, there are usually other psychiatric problems present, although the habit can develop without any other symptoms. Therefore, the definitive diagnosis is made by using the fluid deprivation test. Patients are denied fluid for eight hours. People without diabetes insipidus will then excrete a small amount of concentrated urine, because their bodies will conserve water. People with compulsive water drinking will also be able to concentrate their urine to some degree. However, those with diabetes insipidus cannot conserve water and so will excrete a large amount of dilute urine.

To differentiate between diabetes insipidus caused by damage to the pituitary and that caused by desensitization of the kidney to the actions of ADH, some of the hormone is given to the patient. If the pituitary is the culprit, urine concentrations will rise, whereas if the kidney is desensitized, this will not happen.

TREATMENT

This disease may be treated using a number of different ADH-type drugs. Pitressin tannate-in-oil is injected into the muscle every two to four days. Patients who do not like constant injections can use DDAVP once or twice a day, taken in the form of a nasal inhalant. Lysine vasopressin nasal spray is also very effective, but it must be used every three to six hours.

DIABETES MELLITUS

DEFINITION

Diabetes mellitus is a disease characterized by the inability of the body to produce enough insulin to permit the tissues to absorb glucose from the blood at a sufficiently rapid rate. This results in a failure to provide the body's tissues with the energy they need. A person may be diabetic because the beta cells of the pancreas, which produce insulin, are destroyed. This is called insulin-dependent diabetes (IDD) and mainly develops in children and adults under the age of thirty. On the other hand, diabetes may occur because the person's tissues become resistant to the effects of insulin (meaning that it takes more insulin to permit glucose absorption) and the pancreas just cannot produce enough to compensate for this resistance. This type of the disease is known as non-insulin-dependent diabetes (NIDD) and is most frequently found in middle-aged and older people.

There are also a number of diabetics who do not fit into either category. Some young diabetics get NIDD and in this case the disease is known as maturity onset diabetes of the young (MODY). Conversely, some older people get IDD.

HOW COMMON IS IT?

Diabetes is the most common endocrinological disorder in the world. Approximately 1 percent of the population have it, although in some world groups like those of the Pima Indians in Arizona and the Naruans people of Polynesia, the prevalence is 30 percent or even higher. There are between eleven and twelve million diabetics in America; about 85 percent of them have NIDD.

There is a definite genetic component to this ailment. Fifty percent of the twins of IDDs also develop the disease; 20 percent have a first-degree relative (mother, father, sister, brother) with IDD. It is 12 to 20 percent more common in boys than girls.

The incidence of NIDD increases with age: the majority of people who develop it are in their sixties or seventies. In fact, 2 percent of the population in their seventies have diabetes. Here the disease is more prevalent in women than in men. NIDD also has a genetic component; 25 percent of people with it have a first-degree relative who also suffers from the illness, and almost all identical twins of NIDD sufferers will come down with the disease eventually. NIDD is also much more common in the obese (those who are 10 percent or more overweight).

CAUSES

Insulin-dependent diabetes:

It is believed that people who have IDD are born with genes that make their immune systems work abnormally when assaulted by certain viruses or other environmental toxicants. In response to the attack, especially by the Coxsackie and mumps viruses, their immune systems begin to destroy the body's pancreatic beta cells. This process can take several years.

Non-insulin dependent diabetes:

This type has nothing to do with viruses, although it also seems to be inherited. Here, the person's tissues become less and less responsive to the effects of insulin. Stress, illness, and especially obesity can bring out the disease. Sometimes an obese diabetic can significantly correct his disease by losing all his excess weight.

CASE HISTORY

Helen Gold, a sixty-year-old secretary, had suffered from a weight problem for most of her life. Over the last few months, however, she started losing weight without even trying to and felt unusually fatigued at times. At first she tried to convince herself that the tiredness and weight loss were caused by all the extra work her newly appointed boss was tossing on her desk, but in the back of her mind she knew that this could not explain her constant, intense thirst and need to urinate far more frequently than usual. She remembered the same symptoms in her sister, when she was diagnosed with diabetes several years earlier. When the fatigue and weakness got so bad Helen could no longer work through the day, she went to see her doctor.

The doctor found abnormally high levels of glucose in her urine and suspected diabetes, confirming the diagnosis by giving Helen a blood glucose test. He prescribed an drug called chlorpropamide to be taken by mouth, and told her to watch her diet, particularly limiting her sugar intake. Over the next few weeks he monitored her blood and urine glucose levels but was unable to keep them in the normal range, despite increasing doses of the drug. After two months of therapy, he switched her to a daily dose of insulin to be injected before breakfast. Her blood glucose level dropped to the normal range, she stopped losing weight, and began to feel much better.

SIGNS AND SYMPTOMS

Early Symptoms or Warning Signs:

Frequent urination and a raging thirst; irritation of the genitals; marked loss of weight (mostly in IDD), energy, and strength; slow healing of cuts and bruises; anxiety, sweating and hunger pains three to four hours after eating a heavy meal; dry, itching skin, as well as frequent skin infections.

Long-Term Effects of Diabetes:

Even with medication, it is extremely difficult to keep blood glucose levels in diabetics in the normal range at all times. It is believed that this poor control of blood glucose levels leads to long term side effects, although not all diabetics who have had the illness for a long period of time develop these symptoms. However, the tissue damage resulting from the diabetic condition can affect most of the organ systems of the body.

On the whole, diabetics are more subject to:

- Coronary artery disease and high blood pressure, which can lead to strokes or heart attacks;
- Hardening of the arteries in the legs, especially below the knee, leading to severe pain on walking; as well as dry, hairless skin which can become ulcerative and gangrenous at pressure points (such as where shoes rub against the back of the foot);
- Eye problems, from minor cloudiness of the eye lens to blindness;
- Kidney problems, which can lead to kidney failure;
- Nervous system problems, such as loss of sensation in the hands or feet, sensitive or painful patches of skin, temporary paralysis of certain muscles (including the eye muscle), and less commonly, nerve damage leading to impotence, diarrhea, and an inability to urinate;
- Infections, such as fungal infections of the genital area and feet, urinary tract infections developing into full-blown kidney infections; and tuberculosis.

Hypoglycemia, or abnormally low sugar levels, is a common cause of coma in the diabetic. This usually happens because a meal is missed or too much insulin is taken. All diabetics should learn to recognize the signs of hypoglycemia, because left untreated it can progress to a coma leading to brain and heart damage. Early warning signs include light-headedness or dizziness, sweating, numbness and tingling around the mouth, palpitations, restlessness, weakness, agitation, trembling, headache, depression, fatigue, anxiety, and an inability to concentrate. Diabetics carry glucose tablets with them which they take if they experience these symptoms.

A diabetic coma can arise as a result of hypoglycemia or hyperglycemia. In the first case, there is too little glucose in the blood to supply the tissues with what they need to sustain their energy demands. In the latter case, there is not enough insulin to allow the tissues to absorb the life-sustaining glucose. In both cases this results in the body breaking down fat to supply the tissues with energy. The byproducts of this broken-down fat are called ketone bodies and they make the blood very acidic, causing a coma.

The first signs of a coma are apathy, thirst, and excess urination. Vomiting usually follows. The patient's breathing becomes abnormally heavy and smells of acetone (as in nail polish). He or she will have a rapid pulse, may have severe stomach pains, and if left untreated, will lose consciousness. Such patients require careful medical attention to reduce the acidity of their blood, restore their blood glucose levels to normal with insulin, and replace the body fluids and minerals lost through excess urination.

METHODS OF DIAGNOSIS

The combination of thirst, frequent urination, and loss of weight, together with the presence of glucose in the urine are enough to diagnose diabetes. However, NIDDs may have no symptoms. In these cases, the diagnosis can be confirmed by taking a blood glucose measurement two hours after a meal (which, in the presence of the disease, would be 180 milligrams per 100 milliliters of blood or higher) or by taking a blood glucose measurement after an all-night fast (which in a diabetic would be 120 milligrams per 100 milliliters of blood or higher).

An oral glucose tolerance test is only done when the patient has glucose in the urine but their blood glucose levels are not abnormally high. This test is carried out after the patient has been on a high carbohydrate diet for at least three days. The patient then comes in for the test after an overnight fast. No smoking is allowed during the test. The patient drinks 75 grams of glucose in 300 milliliters of water and blood samples are taken at 0, 60, and 120 minutes. The normal levels for these three times are less than 120 milligram/100 milliliter, 180 milligram/100 milliliter, and 120 milligram/100 milliliter (or below 135 milligram/100 milliliter in the elderly), respectively.

Some patients have an impaired ability to absorb glucose that doesn't quite qualify them as having diabetes. These people may have normal blood glucose levels before taking the glucose tolerance test, but when they receive the glucose in the test, they absorb it more slowly than normal, and so at the 120 minute point their levels will be abnormally high. This group of patients may improve with time, develop diabetes at some later point, or stay the same.

TREATMENT

The purpose of the treatment is to make the body absorb glucose normally, which can be achieved through diet, drugs that stimulate insulin production, drugs that make the tissues more sensitive to the actions of insulin, and insulin.

There are three main types of patients:

- In the obese and mainly middle-aged or elderly diabetics (most NIDDs fall into this group), reducing the caloric and carbohydrate intake is often enough to cause a loss of body weight and complete disappearance of the diabetes. However, the condition usually returns when the person is under stress or falls behind on his diet. Therefore, it is obviously very important for these people to stick to a strict diet. Even specially marketed "diabetic foods" must be restricted as they contain the sugars sorbitol and fructose which are rich in calories. Exercise is also good, since it helps in weight loss as well as makes the tissues more sensitive to insulin. (For all diabetics, twenty minutes or more of vigorous daily exercise can reduce the amount of insulin needed).

- If after two months of restricting the diet, the NIDD or MODY (maturity onset diabetes of the young) still has a high blood glucose level, a drug which lowers blood glucose should be taken.

- Juvenile-onset diabetics with IDD need to follow a diet containing the same amounts of carbohydrates at meals every day, and take insulin to permit glucose absorption.

DIETARY TREATMENT:

Calories: Caloric intake should be aimed at achieving ideal body weight (in the IDD this generally means gaining weight, whereas for the NIDD it means losing weight). Women should estimate their ideal body weight by allowing 100 pounds for the first five feet and five pounds for each additional inch over five feet. In men, 106 pounds should be allowed for the first five feet and six pounds for every inch over that. If a person has a medium or heavy frame, five to ten pounds must also be added. Hence, a man with a medium frame who is six feet tall will have an ideal weight of approximately 183 pounds (106 plus 72 plus 5).

Fat: Fat intake should be limited to 20-30 percent of the total daily calories. This is because diabetes is often associated with high blood fat levels which increase the risk of atherosclerosis (responsible for all the complications of diabetes). The diabetic should adopt a diet low in saturated fat and cholesterol (found in animal products and coconut) and higher in polyunsaturated and monounsaturated fat (found in fish and vegetable products).

Protein: Ideally, a woman needs about 45 grams of protein per day and a man 55 grams a day, which is equal to two to three servings of protein-rich foods such as fish, meat, or dairy products. Diabetics are better off eating fish and poultry, with their lower fat content, as much as they can.

Carbohydrates: The blood glucose level is closely affected by the carbohydrate intake. In diabetics, the amount eaten every day should be kept constant and should depend on the amount of physical activity done by the person. A young active person may need 180 grams of carbohydrate per day, whereas an older sedentary one may only require 100 grams.

Carbohydrates are sugars and come in two forms: simple and complex. Simple sugars include glucose, fructose, sucrose, galactose, and lactose. Complex carbohydrates are mainly starches. Simple sugars are absorbed very rapidly by the body and so will raise blood sugar to high levels. Although all sugars must be converted to glucose in the body, they raise blood sugar levels to different degrees. Of all the simple sugars, fructose (found in fruit) is the best to eat. Sucrose (table sugar) will raise blood glucose levels much more quickly. The more gradual the increase, the easier it is for the diabetic's body to absorb. No more than 10-15 percent of all calories consumed should come from simple sugars of any kind.

Complex carbohydrates are much better, since they take a longer time to be broken down in the digestive system, resulting in a fairly slow absorption and a gradual increase in blood sugar. For this reason, 50-60 percent of dietary calories should come from complex carbohydrates.

Fiber: High fiber diets can cause a slower and more sustained release of glucose from the gastrointestinal tract into the bloodstream, which will prevent wide swings in blood sugar that may occur when simple sugars are taken in the absence of fiber. In addition, the amount of insulin needed to control blood sugar is often reduced by high fiber diets. For this reason, diabetics are advised to eat whole meal bread, bran, beans, vegetables, potato skins, and the skins of fruit.

Meal planning: Meals should be planned carefully. In addition to what is eaten, how often meals are taken is also very important to the diabetic, particularly for the IDDs. Even though modern insulin preparations can release insulin slowly from the injection site, injected insulin cannot mimic the precise and immediate responses of insulin secreted from the pancreas. Therefore, it is very important to avoid periods of feasting (when blood sugar levels may rise too high) or fasting (when blood sugar levels may fall too low). This is best accomplished by eating five or six small meals during the course of the day.

DRUG TREATMENT:

If after two months of sticking to a good diet, the patient with NIDD or MODY still cannot keep his blood glucose at normal levels, he is usually given a drug from the sulfonylurea group, such as tolbutamide, chlorpropamide, acetohexamide, or tolazamide. These drugs act by stimulating the release of insulin by the pancreas and by making the tissues more sensitive to insulin. They can also be too effective and lower blood glucose levels below normal, causing hypoglycemia. They may cause weight gain, as well, which is certainly not desirable for most NIDDs.

Sulfonylureas do not work very well in 25 percent of diabetics and so an alternative group of drugs called biguanides (such as phenformin and metformin) may be used. These increase the sensitivity of the tissues to insulin, making a little bit go a long way, but they do not stimulate the release of insulin by the pancreas. They also decrease appetite and reduce a person's ability to digest food substances. Both factors help to lower weight and so make these the drugs of choice in treating obese NIDDs. These drugs may also be used in conjunction with sulfonyl-ureas. However, they may exacerbate liver, kidney, and cardiovascular diseases and so should not be used in patients with these problems.

All children, young adults (except those with MODY) and those older diabetics who cannot be controlled by diet or sulfonylureas and biguanides need to take insulin. In a person without diabetes, insulin is secreted by the pancreas after blood glucose levels rise following a meal. In order to mimic this pattern of events, insulin injections would have to be given every time the diabetic ate and the amount given would have to be just enough to cause absorption of the carbohydrate content of that meal. But since few people like to inject themselves, and frequent injections are neither acceptable nor very practical, most IDDs spread their carbohydrate intake throughout the day in an even fashion and give themselves two injections of an insulin mixture, one before breakfast and one before the evening meal. Some older people give themselves only one injection before breakfast to cover them for the whole day.

TREATMENT FOR THE LONG-TERM EFFECTS OF DIABETES:
By carefully controlling blood glucose and blood fat levels through diet and medication, as well as by preventing high blood pressure, the development of coronary artery disease can be effectively postponed.

Any infection in the legs is treated with antibiotics to prevent gangrene from setting in. (In fact, any type of physical infections in the diabetic must be attended to immediately.) Close attention must be paid to keeping the feet healthy and scrupulously clean and only comfortable shoes that do not rub the feet or cause corns and other foot problems should be worn. Arterial bypass surgery may be done if there is a blockage in the leg.

Various surgical techniques can be used to minimize eye damage resulting from hemorrhages and scar tissue, and they can improve sight if the problem is caught in its early stages.

NEW FORMS OF TREATMENT:
As mentioned, IDDs appear to suffer from a malfunctioning of the immune system. In France, researchers are now taking advantage of this fact by trying to arrest the disease through the administration of drugs that suppress the immune system. However, such drugs make patients more susceptible to infection, and once the drug is withdrawn, the pancreas begins to deteriorate once again. Future experiments in this field might reveal a way to overcome these problems and effectively treat diabetics in this manner.

EXCESS GROWTH HORMONE
(see Acromegaly)

GIGANTISM
(see Acromegaly)

FAILURE TO MENSTRUATE
(see Amenorrhea)

GYNECOMASTIA

DEFINITION
Gynecomastia is the enlargement of breasts in a man.

HOW COMMON IS IT?
Some type of enlargement of the breasts affects 60 to 70 percent of all boys as they go through puberty. While it usually involves both breasts, it may only affect one. In teenagers, the extra breast tissue usually wastes away without any treatment within a year to a year and a half.

Breast enlargement is also quite common in boys at birth as well as in older men. With these groups and teenagers, the cause is known to be a sex hormone imbalance. But up to one-third of all cases of gynecomastia that do not fall into these three groups have no known cause.

CAUSES
Estrogen and prolactin stimulate breast development in both sexes. Estrogen has the main effect at all times except during pregnancy, when prolactin is of greater importance. Ten percent of the estrogen found in a boy's body is made in the testes; the remaining 90 percent is made in the fat tissue, where testosterone from the testes and androgen from the adrenal glands (androstenedione) are converted into estrogen. However, only a small amount of the testosterone and androstenedione produced in a boy's body is converted to estrogen and the vast majority remains as male sex hormones: so much so in fact that male sex hormones are normally two hundred times the level of estrogen.

If this ratio changes and estrogen levels go up, gynecomastia can occur. This may happen in a number of ways, but most cases occur naturally during the neonatal (after birth) period, adolescence, or old age.

Neonatal gynecomastia: The condition seen in babies is transient and caused by the mother's estrogen moving across the placenta to the baby. Within a short time after birth the problem begins to disappear.

Adolescent gynecomastia: Here the condition is caused by the increased production of estrogen by the testes at puberty. While both estrogen and testosterone are produced by the testes in increasing quantities during this time, the estrogen levels peak before the testosterone levels do and this upsets the normal 200 to 1 ratio. However, testosterone soon catches up in most boys and so the breasts eventually waste away to normal size. If the condition persists beyond the age or sixteen or seventeen the breast tissue may have to be removed surgically.

Gynecomastia in the elderly: From the sixth decade of life onwards the testes produce a little less testosterone and tend to increase the amount converted into estrogen in the fat tissue, which can lead to breast development.

There are other less common causes of gynecomastia. The major one is the use of the medications that either mimic the effects of estrogen or have effects that work against male sex hormones. Such drugs include spironolactone, chemotherapeutic drugs, cimetidine, estrogen, testosterone (because it causes increased conversion to estrogen in the fat tissue), digitalis, digoxin, gonadotropins, methyldopa, phenothiazines, tricyclic antidepressants, cyproterone acetate, ketoconazole, deoxycortisone, marijuana, griseofulvin, and reserpine. However, you should know that just because you are taking one of these drugs it does not mean that you will develop breasts: Only a few people experience this side effect.

In about one in 1000 male births, a condition called Klinefelter's syndrome appears, which is a genetic disorder characterized by underdevelopment of the testes. Because of their reduced testosterone levels, these boys develop gynecomastia.

Ten to 40 percent of young people who suffer from an overactive thyroid gland (hyperthyroidism) produce excess androgens in their adrenal glands, which are turned into estrogens in the fat tissue and can cause gynecomastia. Men with chronic liver or kidney disease can also develop breasts because such illnesses stimulate the hypothalamus to produce excess prolactin. Men in the twenty to forty-five age range with estrogen-secreting tumors of the testes or adrenal glands can also develop breasts. The condition may appear because of other tumors that produce gonadotropins (which stimulate the testes to produce more estrogen and/or testosterone) such as tumors of the lungs, testes, and liver.

Finally, sometimes a man who is gaining weight rapidly after severe weight loss (such as following a serious illness) can develop breasts.

CASE HISTORY

John G. was a thirty-four-year-old bachelor and loving every minute of it. He enjoyed the singles scene and frequently took out pretty young women. But suddenly, almost out of the blue, his interest in sex began to decrease. Although he made jokes about it, he was worried. He hoped he wasn't getting old before his time.

A few months later, John noticed his breasts were starting to grow larger and were quite tender to the touch. Throughout the day he was aware of his shirt rubbing against them. As they grew even more, he panicked. He went to see his family doctor who referred him to an endocrinologist.

The specialist questioned John about his drinking habits. Since John didn't drink to excess the doctor knew his decreased sexual libido wasn't caused by alcohol consumption. John also said that he took no medications and didn't smoke marijuana.

While examining John, the doctor noticed that his skin was very fine to the touch—indicative of an estrogen excess—and that his right testis was significantly smaller than his left one. Suspecting a tumor, the doctor did a number of tests and found that John's body was producing abnormal amounts of estrogen.

John was scheduled for exploratory surgery, where an estrogen-secreting tumor was found on his left testis and removed. John was given irradiation treatment after surgery and completely recovered. His enlarged breasts disappeared. Then he had himself checked for fertility and was found to be normal. Two years later, John met a very special woman at a friend's party. They were married shortly afterwards and now have two healthy children.

SIGNS AND SYMPTOMS

Enlargement of one or both breasts. It is rarely painful, although sometimes the breast tissue becomes quite tender (especially when it occurs in men who develop breasts because of taking certain drugs).

METHODS OF DIAGNOSIS

The first thing the doctor does is to distinguish between gynecomastia and the enlargement of the breasts caused by being overweight, where extra fat is laid down in the breast area. Gynecomastia is found by pressing down on the area. Fat is soft, whereas gynecomastia causes the tissue to become hard under the nipple.

The next thing to consider is the age of the male. If he is around fourteen and the breasts have developed from the time he went into puberty then there is usually nothing to worry about. However, if the condition is appearing in a thirty-year-old man there may be a serious medical problem involved, such as a tumor. If the condition is of long standing, the man has little interest in sex, has abnormally small testes, and lacks some or all of the usual male characteristics (a beard, hairiness of the limbs and chest, a deep voice, an enlarged Adam's apple), he could be suffering from Klinefelter's syndrome, which can be diagnosed with a chromosome test.

If a man has only one enlarged breast and either a bloody discharge from the nipple, or one or more immobile lumps or a lump in the armpit, then breast cancer may be present and the proper tests are carried out. The presence of one small or normal-sized testis and one enlarged testis often denotes a tumor in the enlarged testis.

Various tests can be done on a patient with gynecomastia. In adults, a chest X-ray will pick up any lung tumors. Blood tests for LH levels, HCG (human chorionic gonadotropin—the gonadotropin produced by tumors), testosterone levels, and other androgen, estrogen, and prolactin levels may be carried out. The urine can then be analyzed for estrogen and substances called 17-ketosteroids (which are the breakdown products of adrenal steroids and are in abnormally high concentrations if there is an adrenal tumor).

TREATMENT

In the case of an adolescent or baby, the breasts will usually get smaller again and go back to normal. Slightly enlarged breasts in the elderly may be left untreated if there is no serious disorder present and if the patient is not seriously upset by the condition. When drugs are the cause, they can be discontinued and an alternate medication found. If tumors are the culprit, they are removed. When the condition is persistent in adolescents, antiestrogen drugs such as tamoxifen or clomiphene, or weak androgens such as danazol can be prescribed, but they should be given within a year of the appearance of the enlarged breasts (in order to work most effectively) and should not be continued for longer than six months, as they may interfere with normal development. If gynecomastia had been caused by hyperthyroidism, antithyroid drugs or radioactive iodine may be used.

A mammectomy (removal of the breast) may be done surgically in cases where the added tissue does not normally shrink, such as in the elderly and in some adolescents, and especially if the breasts are painful or cosmetically disturbing. Sometimes dihydrotestosterone (a potent form of testosterone) is mixed with a gelatin-like substance and placed over the breast area for six hours. This causes the breast to shrink in some patients.

HIRSUTISM

DEFINITION
Hirsutism is the word used to describe excess body hair in women. This hair is grown in androgen-sensitive areas, or in other words, where men are more prone to growing hair (face, chin, neck, chest, and so forth).

HOW COMMON IS IT?
One in eighty women have some form of hirsutism. It is found more frequently among Caucasians than among other races: it is more common in darkly pigmented Caucasians from Mediterranean countries and the Middle East than in Nordic females. Oriental, American Indian, and black women rarely have the condition. In addition, hirsutism tends to increase after menopause and runs in families.

CAUSES
Over 90 percent of all women suffering from hirsutism have high androgen levels. Of all the androgens it is primarily testosterone that stimulates this kind of hair growth and so its production is increased in nearly all hirsute females. Testosterone is produced from three sources: 25 percent comes from the ovaries; 25 percent from the adrenal glands; and 50 percent comes from fat and muscle tissue, made from other androgens secreted by the adrenal glands and ovaries. Almost all of the testosterone in the woman's body (97-99 percent) circulates in the blood bound to proteins, of which the most important one is sex

hormone binding globulin (SHBG). It is the small amount of remaining unbound testosterone which is free to act on the tissues and cause conditions like hirsutism.

Therefore, in most hirsute women, SHBG levels are reduced (leaving less testosterone bound), and although total testosterone levels may be normal, the concentration of the free hormone is increased. Women who have these types of hormonal readings usually have a family history of hirsutism. However, everything else about them is normal, they have regular menstrual periods, and they show no signs of increased masculinity (lowered voice, loss of body curves). Women with these characteristics are said to have idiopathic or constitutional hirsutism, which is believed to be caused by an increased sensitivity of the hair follicles to androgens.

Other hirsute women have irregular and infrequent menstrual periods in addition to abnormal hair growth. In these women, the ovaries contain many cysts and produce more androgens and less estrogen than normal. This condition is called polycystic ovarian disease (PCOD) or Stein Leventhal syndrome, and its cause is unknown. Such women are often infertile due to infrequent ovulation and may also be obese. Almost half (40 percent) of the women with this disease inherit it.

In addition to idiopathic hirsutism and PCOD there are other causes of hirsutism that are more rare such as Cushing's Syndrome (discussed in the Guide). Also, masculinizing tumors of the ovary or adrenal glands are suspected when the hirsutism develops quickly and severely and is accompanied by balding, shrinking (atrophy) of the breasts, development of an Adam's apple, deepening of the voice, increased muscular structure, loss of body contours, acne, and enlargement of the clitoris—all traits of what is known as virilization, or becoming more like a man.

Hirsutism can develop during pregnancy because of androgens produced by the placenta. During menopause, some of the short, fine, downy hair that covers parts of the woman's body may become darkly pigmented and coarse because of an increase in ovarian androgen secretion. Hirsutism may also be caused by a number of drugs, such as dilantin, androgens, diazoxide, and minoxidil.

CASE HISTORY

Maria Denucci, a twenty-year-old secretary for a publishing company, began to grow excess hair on her face. In the last year, she had missed six periods and gained fifteen pounds, despite the fact that her eating habits and lifestyle had remained the same. She had even stopped taking birth control pills six months earlier in an attempt to lose weight. Maria was also very depressed and had lost her usually healthy interest in sex.

When the hair on her face started to increase and become unsightly, she consulted her doctor. He found no obvious evidence of virilization. He then took a blood sample and found that her testosterone levels were mildly elevated. An ultrasound test showed that both ovaries were enlarged. The doctor suspected PCOD. His diagnosis was confirmed when he measured her LH levels after giving her an injection of LH releasing hormone. The LH measurements rose to way above normal values.

The doctor treated Maria by giving her an oral contraceptive. After three months the doctor again tested her testosterone levels to find that they were now normal. The medication was continued and within twelve months she had lost the unsightly hair, the extra weight, and felt fine again.

SIGNS AND SYMPTOMS

Excessive hair growth in one or more of the following areas: the upper lip, the sideburns, the chin, the neck, the chest, the lower abdomen (in a line approaching upwards from the pubic region toward the belly button), between the legs, and over the limbs.

METHODS OF DIAGNOSIS

Since most of the women with this condition are suffering from idiopathic hirsutism, the main objective of the physician is to distinguish between this and other types of hirsutism.

In idiopathic hirsutism, there is often a family history of the disorder among the female relatives. The age of onset and evidence of virilization are also important clues to the cause of the condition. Idiopathic hirsutism starts at puberty or in the early teens, progresses slowly from that point onwards, and is not accompanied by abnormal menstruation. PCOD starts at the same time but is accompanied by menstrual abnormalities and even amenorrhea (loss of menstrual periods). If the hirsutism begins suddenly (often several years after menopause), it usually suggests an androgen-secreting tumor on the ovary or adrenal gland. If virilization is present, either an androgen-secreting tumor or severe PCOD could be the cause.

In addition to a physical examination and a family history, the doctor may also take a number of blood tests. The testosterone circulating in the blood as well as adrenal androgens are usually measured. In many cases of either PCOD or idiopathic hirsutism one or both will be higher than normal. Very high levels of testosterone might mean an androgen-secreting tumor in the ovaries or adrenal glands. Modern scanning techniques such as ultrasound and CAT scans are useful for differentiating between PCOD and tumors. In PCOD both ovaries will be enlarged. It is highly unlikely, on the other hand, that a woman will have tumors in both ovaries, so women with androgen-producing tumors will usually show one enlarged ovary. If PCOD is suspected, LH levels are measured by giving an injection of LH releasing hormone. When a woman has PCOD, these levels will rise to a higher than normal value.

Other causes of hirsutism, such as Cushing's syndrome may be easily diagnosed from their other symptoms (see Cushing's syndrome in the Guide).

TREATMENT

Hirsutism may be treated by various combinations of antiandrogens (for severe cases) and cosmetic therapy.

Idiopathic hirsutism: This is often treated with birth control pills. The estrogen they contain decreases the amount of testosterone in the bloodstream. Estrogen also increases the serum hormone binding globulin (SHBG) which lowers the amount of free testosterone in the body by binding to more of it. The reduced testosterone levels decrease the rate of hair growth and reduce the coarseness of the hair. It takes about nine months of estrogen therapy before significant improvement can be seen.

Cosmetic measures are also important for reducing the hirsutism. Unwanted hair may be removed by tweezing, waxing, bleaching, chemical depilatories, shaving, and electrolysis. Shaving is the safest method but electrolysis is the only permanent way of removing the hair. Incidentally, shaving does not increase hair growth or the thickness of the hair shaft.

Polycystic ovarian disease (PCOD): As described in the case history, birth control pills are also used to treat this group of hirsute patients. The pills of choice are Ortho-Novum 2 mg and Demulen. After nine months of treatment some improvement can be expected. Cosmetic therapy is also very useful for these women. In addition, because many of them do not ovulate, they must be medicated with clomiphene (Clomid, Serophene), which induces ovulation, if they want to become pregnant.

Other forms of hirsutism such as tumors, Cushing's Syndrome, drug-induced hirsutism: Removal of the cause usually leads to regression of the hirsutism.

HYPERPARATHYROIDISM

DEFINITION

Hyperparathyroidism is the overactivity of the parathyroid glands. These are four glands that sit behind the thyroid gland, two on each side. They secrete parathyroid hormone (PTH) which regulates blood calcium levels. When these levels go down, PTH is secreted, causing the extraction of calcium from the bone, an increase in calcium absorption by the intestines, and boosting the role of the kidneys in helping to maintain blood calcium levels. Conversely, when these levels rise, PTH secretion is inhibited. In hyperparathyroidism, PTH is secreted in abnormally large amounts causing high blood calcium levels and gradual weakening of the bones.

HOW COMMON IS IT?

One in 800 people over the age of twenty have this disease, which is three times more common in women. Most patients are over forty years old.

CAUSES

In 85 percent of all cases, the disorder is caused by a benign tumor (called an adenoma) which produces large amounts of PTH. Most of the other cases are caused by an overgrowth of the parathyroid glands, and in rare instances parathyroid cancer is the problem.

CASE HISTORY

Gertrude Mitchnik, seventy, a retired lawyer, went to see her doctor because of severe pain in her right knee. This was really the last straw for her in a long line of annoying symptoms that had been appearing recently for no apparent reason. Over the last three months, Gertrude, an active senior citizen who normally saw her doctor only once a year for a checkup, had been suffering from a great deal of bone pain, a lack of her usual healthy appetite, occasional vomiting, fatigue upon any kind of exertion, and frequent urination.

Gertrude's doctor admitted her to the hospital where he did a whole battery of tests and x-rays. He found that she had arthritis in her knee, high blood and urine calcium levels, and low blood phosphorus levels. His diagnosis of hyperparathyroidism was confirmed when her blood PTH levels were also found to be high.

Exploratory surgery was done on Gertrude's neck and an adenoma on one of the parathyroid glands was found. It was removed. One week later Gertrude went home, feeling much better.

SIGNS AND SYMPTOMS

Patients with mild cases are unlikely to show any symptoms and the presence of the disease is detected only if their doctor screens their blood for calcium in the course of doing other diagnostic tests. Patients with a more severe case of the disease will have very high calcium levels in their blood, which leads to lethargy, fatigue, weakness, loss of appetite, nausea, vomiting, constipation, thirst, and frequent urination. If the blood calcium levels become extremely high the person becomes drowsy and confused. Since many people do not consult their doctors until they have had this problem for some time, they can suffer from complications such as kidney stones and the severe pain associated with them, back pain, blood in the urine, or peptic ulcers. Some patients develop the type of arthritis characterized by calcium deposits in the joints.

METHODS OF DIAGNOSIS

A person with a history of high blood calcium levels for over a year, who has not suffered any type of weight loss or other symptoms of malignancy does not suffer from the main cause of high blood calcium levels—namely, cancer. The diagnosis of hyperparathyroidism can be confirmed by measuring PTH levels. X-rays may show kidney stones and erosions of the bones in the hands. Other characteristics of patients with this disease include low blood phosphorus levels and high calcium levels in the urine.

TREATMENT

The only effective treatment for hyperparathyroidism is surgery to remove the adenoma or the enlarged gland. Most patients are then discharged, cured of their pain by the second or third day after the operation. Other symptoms quickly disappear.

HYPERTHYROIDISM

DEFINITION

Hyperthyroidism results from the overproduction of thyroid hormones (T3 and T4). The excess hormones cause all reactions in the body to speed up, and are responsible for many unpleasant symptoms, including a gradual loss of weight.

HOW COMMON IS IT?

As many as 2 to 5 people out of 1000 have this disease. The majority of patients are female and most are in the twenty- to forty-year-old age group, although it can occur at any age.

CAUSES

There are three main causes of hyperthyroidism:

- Grave's Disease
  This type of hyperthyroidism accounts for 80 percent of all cases, tends to affect young women (the female to male ratio is 7 or 8 to 1), and runs in families. It is caused by the patient's own immune system, which produces antibodies that stimulate the thyroid gland to continuously produce thyroid hormones. (In a person with normal thyroid function, the gland will only produce hormones when stimulated to do so by TSH, which is released by the pituitary gland.) Graves' disease is another autoimmune illness.

- Toxic Multinodular Goiter (Plummer's Disease)
  This ailment accounts for 10 percent of all cases of hyperthyroidism and is generally found in older people (typically women over the age of sixty). In these patients, discrete areas of the thyroid gland swell to form nodules (lumps) in the neck area, instead of the whole gland expanding and causing a smooth swelling or goiter in the neck. The lumps begin to produce thyroid hormones even when there is no stimulation by TSH. If enough of these

lumps produce excess hormone, there will be too much T3 and T4 in the body, resulting in hyperthyroidism. No one yet knows precisely what causes the development of these lumps.

- Toxic Adenoma
  This is responsible for about 5 percent of patients with hyperthyroid conditions, and here one nodule slowly grows and produces more and more thyroid hormone until it causes hyperthyroidism. By the time the disease develops, the nodule is usually larger than one and a half inches in diameter. Toxic adenoma is more commonly found in women, and can occur at any age.

Hyperthyroidism can be caused by outside factors. A person who takes thyroid hormones to treat hypothyroidism may be given too high a dose. Also, as an aftermath of certain illnesses (such as respiratory disease), the thyroid can release large quantities of stored hormones, resulting in a temporary case of hyperthyroidism.

CASE HISTORY
    A young public relations executive named Joan Beresford had been suffering from weakness, nervousness, and an unexplained weight loss for the past six months. She also noticed palpitations whenever she exerted herself, along with an excessive amount of perspiration even when she sat in air conditioned rooms. In fact, she would sometimes feel so hot at night that she couldn't bear to sleep under any kind of cover. Her eyes felt sandy and watery, and her periods became irregular. A co-worker suggested that her loss of weight, despite the fact that she seemed to be eating even more than usual, might be a symptom of some serious illness and so a worried Joan went to see her doctor.
    The doctor first noticed that Joan's eyes bulged and when he asked her to look down, her eyelids did not follow the eyeballs. Her thyroid gland was also enlarged and smooth. When asked to stretch out her hands, they trembled noticeably, and an examination of her fingers showed slight clubbing. The doctor therefore suspected Graves' disease and upon taking a blood sample and analyzing it for T3 and T4 levels found them both to be abnormally high, confirming his diagnosis. Joan was first given a drug called propranolol to control her symptoms, along with an antithyroid drug called methimazole, which brought her hyperthyroidism under control within a few weeks. At that point, the

propranolol was discontinued and the dose of methimazole was reduced. After a further eighteen months on that drug, it was withdrawn, because Joan, like many other patients, was found to have gone into remission. She has not taken any medication for two years now and so far has not suffered from any recurrences.

SIGNS AND SYMPTOMS
These are wide ranging and include:
- Intolerance to heat;
- Agitation and irritability;
- Excessive perspiration;
- Palpitations (rapid heart beats);
- Diarrhea or loose stools;
- Weight loss despite an increased appetite and food intake;
- Weakness and fatigue;
- Loss of muscle mass and strength;
- Irregular or absent menstrual periods;
- Impotence or gynecomastia in the male (both discussed in the Guide);
- Warm hands that tend to shake when outstretched;
- Shortness of breath;
- Nervousness, restlessness and anxiety;
- Smooth, velvety skin;
- Clubbing of the fingers and toes;
- Swollen shins;
- Sore, watery, and bulging eyes;
- Failure of the lids of the eyes to follow the eye downwards when the patient looks down (so one can see the whites of the person's eyes);
- Separation of the nails from the underlying tissue by an accumulation of dead skin; and
- Finer hair that is less curly and tends to fall out;

In the elderly, many of these symptoms may not appear and what one sees instead are only the heart problems, weight loss, weakness, and a loss of appetite. Also, the different causes of hyperthyroidism are marked by specific symptoms (see Methods of Diagnosis).

METHODS OF DIAGNOSIS

The presence of the signs and symptoms mentioned above is usually enough to diagnose the disease, but it is always confirmed by taking a blood sample that is analyzed for T3 and T4 levels. In the hyperthyroid patient, both levels are usually elevated.

The doctor can also distinguish between the different types of hyperthyroidism. In patients with Graves' disease, the goiter will be smooth and there may also be a series of fine vibrations (like pulses) within it, which the doctor can feel when he examines the neck. Young women are generally affected by this ailment and will show the eye but not the heart symptoms. They may also have clubbing of their fingers and toes and the shins may be swollen, with the overlying skin thickened, red, and puckered.

People suffering from Plummer's disease will generally be older and the goiter will feel irregular, with several lumps apparent within the thyroid tissue. They will often have an irregular heartbeat but rarely any eye symptoms or swelling of the shins. With toxic adenoma, there will be one large lump present in the thyroid and other symptoms similar to those of Plummer's disease.

TREATMENT

When a person is first diagnosed with hyperthyroidism due to Graves' disease, he is given propranolol, which alleviates many of the symptoms (including palpitations, shaking, sweating, heat intolerance, and anxiety) within one to two days. The patient is also prescribed a drug that prevents the thyroid gland from producing thyroid hormone, such as methimazole or propylthiouracil. When the thyroid is brought under control, usually after six weeks of treatment, the propranolol is withdrawn and the dose of methimazole or propylthiouracil reduced. The antithyroid drug is then withdrawn completely after the patient's thyroid has been kept at a normal level for twelve to eighteen months. After this time, most patients with Graves' disease go into remission, although approximately half of them do have a relapse and need a second series of treatments with an antithyroid drug. This is the treatment of choice for younger people, pregnant women, and nursing mothers, even though there are some side effects, with skin rashes being the most commonly seen (in five percent of patients; other side effects may include joint pain, jaundice, and problems with the immune system).

Relapsed patients with Graves' disease and patients with nodules may be controlled by the removal of part of their thyroid gland (called a partial thyroidectomy) by a qualified surgeon. Ninety-five percent of patients receiving this treatment gain relief from the condition; 20 percent develop hypothyroidism; and 25 percent are left with an altered vocal quality due to damage to the nerves of the larynx.

Radioactive iodine therapy is an alternative treatment frequently used in patients over the age of forty and in those who have not responded to antithyroid drugs. It can be done on an outpatient basis, is safe, easy, and almost always effective. Radioactive iodine can be given by mouth or as an injection and is rapidly absorbed by the thyroid gland. As the gland takes in the iodine it becomes exposed to an enormous amount of radioactivity, which over a period of three to four months destroys significant quantities of thyroid tissue. In one-third of all cases, the patient is still hyperthyroid six to twelve months after this treatment and needs a second dose. Fifteen percent of patients receiving this kind of therapy develop hypothyroidism within a year and a further three percent develop hypothyroidism each year after that. This is not considered a medical mistake, as it is very difficult to calculate exactly the right amount of radioactive iodine needed to destroy enough thyroid tissue to normalize the patient. Furthermore, the treatment of hypothyroidism is easy, since it only necessitates taking a pill every day.

On the other hand, the fact that radioactive iodine gives off high doses of radiation to the whole body as it travels through the bloodstream means that it should not be given to young people of childbearing age as it could adversely affect the reproductive organs.

Patients over forty with multinodular goiter or toxic adenoma are treated with radioactive iodine and if the goiter is particularly large, with surgery, as spontaneous remission in these cases rarely occurs with the use of antithyroid drugs. For those under forty, surgery is the treatment of choice.

Eye problems (ophthalmopathy) associated with Graves' disease can be unpleasant and difficult to treat but will spontaneously improve over months or years once the thyroid condition is under control.

Swollen shins (called pretibial myxedema) often respond to topical treatment with corticosteroids but will also improve in time once the thyroid condition is under control.

HYPOPARATHYROIDISM

DEFINITION
This disease is characterized by low blood levels of parathyroid hormone which cause low blood calcium levels.

HOW COMMON IS IT?
One out of fifty people who have operations on their thyroid glands get the disease. Rarely, children are born without parathyroid glands and so have the disease. One in 50,000 people (especially women) develop it.

CAUSES
The most common cause of hypoparathyroidism is surgical damage done to the glands during thyroid or other neck operations. Some people (under the age of fifteen) develop the disease when their own immune systems destroy the parathyroid glands (called idiopathic hypoparathyroidism); they often have other autoimmune ailments as well, such as severe anemia and Hashimoto's disease (see Hypothyroidism in the Guide).

CASE HISTORY
A fifty-year-old homemaker named Grace Treadway was found to have low blood calcium and phosphate levels when she went for her annual checkup. Her only complaint was of an occasional tingling in her lips and fingertips when she was tired. She told her doctor that sixteen years ago she had had most of her thyroid gland removed because of cancer. Since her doctor suspected hypoparathyroidism, he ordered a blood PTH test. The level was found to be so low it was almost undetectable, confirming his suspicions.
Grace was treated with vitamin D and calcium supplements and her blood calcium levels checked every one to two months in order to make sure that they did rise too much, due to taking an excessive amount of vitamin D. Grace no longer feels any tingling in her lips or fingers.

SIGNS AND SYMPTOMS
Many patients with the disease do not show any symptoms, whereas others exhibit quite dramatic signs due to the low blood calcium levels, which make the nerves hyperactive. These include:
• Tingling in the face and/or fingers;

- Muscle cramps (in some cases to such a degree that the muscle becomes totally immobile; this is known as tetany);
- Psychoses;
- Convulsions;
- Facial twitching (when the doctor taps lightly on the facial nerve, which crosses the cheek horizontally from the middle of the ear);
- Hand muscles that go into spasm (when the doctor inflates a blood pressure cuff around the arm for three minutes), causing the wrist to flex and the fingers to bunch up;
- Dry and scaly skin;
- Hair that falls out in patches all over the scalp;
- Brittle nails that are prone to fungal infections;
- Cataracts; and
- in children with developing teeth, the enamel does not form properly and is susceptible to decay.

METHODS OF DIAGNOSIS

Analysis of the blood will reveal a low calcium level and a high phosphate level. The EKG (electrocardiogram) is abnormal in people with idiopathic hypoparathyroidism. Those who have the disease because of surgical damage or removal have low blood phosphate levels, which further distinguishes them from the idiopathic patients.

TREATMENT

People with this disease are treated with calcium and vitamin D supplements. The vitamin D increases the absorption of calcium from the digestive tract and is effective in increasing blood calcium to normal levels. However, the blood must be checked regularly to make sure that these levels do not go too high.

HYPOPITUITARISM

DEFINITION

This is a disorder where the pituitary gland is unable to produce enough of one or more of its hormones.

HOW COMMON IS IT?

Approximately 1 in 5000 people suffer from this disorder.

CAUSES

A poorly functioning pituitary may be the result of a variety of causes. It can happen when part of the gland is destroyed by surgery or radiation therapy for a tumor within the pituitary. Prolonged treatment with steroids can suppress the production of the hormone ACTH by the pituitary. Tumors in the gland itself or in surrounding areas of the brain may be responsible, as well as hemorrhages in the brain.

Sometimes pituitary tissue can be destroyed when a woman gives birth and this condition is known as Sheehan's syndrome. The gland always enlarges during pregnancy. If there is a hemorrhage in the birth canal at birth or just prior to birth, it shocks the body and in a few women the arteries supplying the anterior pituitary go into spasm and cut off the blood supply to the front of the gland. While the posterior pituitary has a much better blood supply, it can also be affected; diabetes insipidus (discussed in the Guide), caused by an inadequate amount of the hormone vasopressin (otherwise known as ADH) which is released by the posterior pituitary, does commonly occur in women with Sheehan's syndrome. This syndrome can also develop in men after a severe hemorrhage.

The other causes of hypopituitarism include: damage caused by X-rays of the head, various infections including tuberculosis, fungal infections, syphilis, the blocking of arteries supplying the pituitary with blood due to atherosclerosis, an injury to the base of the skull damaging the pituitary, and disorders of the hypothalamus.

CASE HISTORY

Janine Williams, thirty, hemorrhaged very badly after giving birth to her son Sean two years ago. She was unable to nurse her new baby and had not had a period since her pregnancy. In addition, her breasts became even smaller than they were before she was pregnant. Since Janine wanted another child, she went to see an endocrinologist. He found that her pulse rate was slow, her thyroid gland had shrunk so much he could not feel it when he examined her neck, her uterus was small and her ovaries were also quite shrunken in size. Janine's nipples were pale and she had almost no hair under her arms or in the pubic area.

The doctor measured her blood levels of TSH, cortisol, LH, FSH, and estrogen and found them all to be way below normal. He then did an insulin tolerance test and found that very little growth hormone or ACTH appeared in the blood. He went on to test her with TRH and found that this did not cause the normal rise in TSH levels.

He diagnosed Janine as having hypopituitarism. Although her medical history suggested a classic case of Sheehan's syndrome, he did a CAT scan just to make absolutely certain that she did not have a tumor of the pituitary or related body structures. Fortunately she did not. Janine was treated with FSH, estrogen, cortisol, and thyroid hormone and soon began to have regular periods and feel much better. Almost two years after starting treatment, Janine became pregnant and later gave birth to a healthy baby girl.

SIGNS AND SYMPTOMS

Hypopituitarism caused by Sheehan's syndrome becomes very obvious right away because the woman who has it cannot nurse her newborn infant. This is because her body lacks the pituitary hormone oxytocin, which is responsible for expelling milk from the breast. With other forms of the disease, the onset is often slow and hardly noticeable at first. The symptoms a person begins to exhibit depends on which pituitary hormones are missing. The hormone usually lost first is growth hormone, followed by the gonadotropins (FSH and LH), TSH, and then ACTH.

Growth hormone deficiency cannot be seen easily in adults, but in children a lack of this hormone leads to stunted growth. FSH and LH deficiency leads to: a loss of the sex drive in both men and women; amenorrhea in women; impotence in men; the loss of pubic, body, face and armpit hair; atrophy of the breasts and testicles; infertility; and fine wrinkles at the corners of the mouth and eyes. The loss of FSH and LH also delays sexual development in children.

A lack of TSH leads to intolerance to the cold, a lack of energy, problems in concentrating, and a slowed heart rate. A deficiency of ACTH reduces the activity of the adrenal gland; the resulting lack of cortisol leads to weakness and low blood sugar levels. It can also cause pale, smooth, baby-like skin, and pale nipples. The loss of androgens made by the adrenal gland leads to an absence of sexual drive and of armpit hair in women.

Patients with pituitary hormone deficiencies may also have a loss of vision caused by a tumor in or near the gland.

METHODS OF DIAGNOSIS

Pituitary hormone deficiencies in children can usually be diagnosed easily because the child fails to grow or fails to enter puberty.

If a woman continues to get her menstrual period or a man enjoys normal potency and has normal blood levels of testosterone, hypopituitarism can be ruled out. But the gland must be investigated further if there is any evidence of gonadotropin deficiency.

A lack of the pituitary hormone ADH will prevent the body from concentrating the urine and so the urine will be very dilute first thing in the morning, when it would normally be the most concentrated. The doctor will test the urine in the morning to see whether or not it is dilute.

Measurements of LH, FSH, TSH, ACTH, growth hormone, and prolactin can be done on the blood as well as tests for the hormones produced when the pituitary hormones stimulate their target organs. As you may remember, these pituitary hormones are secreted in the blood and circulate to various organs, which they in turn stimulate. LH and FSH stimulate the sex organs to produce sex hormones; TSH stimulates the thyroid gland to secrete thyroid hormones; ACTH stimulates the adrenal gland to secrete cortisol; and growth hormone stimulates the liver to release glucose. Therefore, by testing the blood for the hormonal levels of these target organs, the doctor can find out exactly how well the pituitary is doing its many jobs throughout the body.

Patients whose pituitary is not producing any or most of its hormones will be diagnosed when their blood tests show low levels of these hormones. Lesser degrees of hypopituitarism can only be found with more sensitive tests called "dynamic" or "stress" tests. One such test is the insulin tolerance test. Here the patient is injected intravenously with insulin. Within thirty minutes blood glucose levels will drop to a very low point, causing the patient to sweat heavily and become very restless. Such a reduction in glucose would cause a normal pituitary to secrete growth hormone and ACTH in large amounts, since both of them raise blood glucose levels and can correct the abnormality. If blood tests do not show a dramatic rise in these hormones after the glucose levels drop, there is evidence of a poorly functioning pituitary. Other "dynamic" tests include injecting TRF and GnRH which should raise the levels in the body of TSH, and FSH and LH, respectively. Again, if this does not happen, there is something wrong with the pituitary gland.

TREATMENT

The treatment of hypopituitarism includes taking care of the cause whenever possible, along with replacing the hormones that are in short supply. Children with growth hormone deficiency are given the hormone, while adults are not. FSH or HCG (human chorionic gonadotropin) are given to stimulate the production of sex hormones and restore fertility in both sexes. In addition, many of these patients also need supplements of sex hormones (estrogen, testosterone, and so forth). The lack of ACTH is corrected by giving cortisol; since cortisol levels are high in the morning and low at night, two doses are given each day, with twice as much taken in the morning as at night, and an additional supplement recommended when the person is under stress (because cortisol helps the body function normally under stressful conditions). Thyroid hormone (T4) is given to compensate for the lack of TSH.

HYPOTHYROIDISM

DEFINITION

Hypothyroidism is a disease in which the thyroid hormones do not carry out their normal functions in the body. In almost all the cases, it develops when the thyroid gland produces insufficient amounts of thyroid hormone to maintain normal blood levels, but in some rare cases it can be caused by a failure of the part of the tissues to respond to normal or even raised levels of thyroid hormones. Because these hormones have such widespread effects on the growth and development of the body, as well as on the workings of all the body's cells, a deficiency can lead to many health problems, ranging from mental retardation in infants to heart failure in adults.

HOW COMMON IS IT?

One in every 1000 men and 2 in every 100 women have the disease. One in 1500 children under the age of twenty have it, and 1 in 5000 infants are born with it.

CAUSES

Hypothyroidism can be caused by a variety of conditions. The most common one involves an inability of the thyroid gland to produce enough hormone because there is too little active tissue present, or because the tissue present cannot make enough. It can also result from a disease of the pituitary that prevents it from producing TSH or a disease of the hypothalamus that prevents it from producing TRH.

In most cases of hypothyroidism, the thyroid gland grows because of the influence of TSH, which is produced in increasing amounts as the level of thyroid hormone in the blood decreases. This is because the body is trying to compensate for the reduced production of thyroid hormone by stimulating the growth of the thyroid tissue. The enlargement of the thyroid gland is known as goiter.

Hashimoto's thyroiditis (found most often in middle-aged women) is accompanied by goiter. A patient with Hashimoto's disease develops hypothyroidism because she produces antibodies that destroy her own thyroid tissue. Diseases of this kind, where the patient destroys part of his or her own body, are called autoimmune diseases.

The use of certain drugs can also lead to hypothyroidism. Lithium carbonate, used in the treatment of manic depression, inhibits the release of thyroid hormone and can cause goiter. People with chronic respiratory infections, who consume excessive quantities of iodine through taking expectorants containing potassium iodide, can cause goiter by inhibiting thyroid hormone manufacture and release in ways not yet clearly understood. (However, as you will see below, everyone needs 150 micrograms of iodine per day to keep the thyroid operating correctly. With iodine, as with most things, the key is moderation.) Other goiter-causing drugs include: cobalt, perchlorates, thiocyanates, thiouracils, carbimazole, resorcinol, para-aminosalicylic acid, and phenylbutazone.

Certain foods contain substances called goitrogens, which prevent the thyroid gland from producing its hormones and can cause hypothyroidism if eaten in excess. In patients with hypothyroidism, goitrogens will exacerbate the condition and make it necessary for these patients to take more thyroid medication. Foods containing goitrogens include: brussels sprouts, cabbage, cassava (from which tapioca pudding is made), cauliflower, kale, kelp, peaches, pears, rutabagas, soybeans, spinach, and turnips. However, cooking destroys the goitrogens in these foods and if enough iodine is consumed each day—by eating foods such as seafood, kelp, cheese, meat, and vegetables—the body is protected against goitrogen-induced hypothyroidism.

Severe iodine deficiency (below fifty micrograms/day) can also cause hypothyroidism. While this is rare in the United States, it is more common in mountainous areas where there is no iodine in the soil such as the Himalayas, Andes, Papua-New Guinea, and Zaire.

Approximately 20 percent of all patients treated for hyperthyroidism (an overactive thyroid) by surgical removal of part of the gland become hypothyroid; nearly 80 percent of hyperthyroid patients treated with radioactive iodine become hypothyroid within fifteen years of treatment.

With infant hypothyroidism, 75 percent of all cases are caused by a failure of the thyroid gland to develop properly and 20 percent are due to a lack of the necessary enzymes to produce thyroid hormone. (The latter condition may also develop in adults, but it is very rare.) The remaining cases of infant hypothyroidism are caused by antithyroid drugs taken by the mother during pregnancy and passing across to the infant while it is in the womb, or by severe iodine deficiency in the mother.

CASE HISTORY

Bette Green, a fifty-nine-year-old homemaker, was suffering from a variety of unusual symptoms that began almost two years before. She complained of increasing tiredness, constipation, muscle weakness and stiffness, and seemed to suffer from the effects of cold weather more than she normally did. She noticed that her skin and hair were excessively dry, her hair was thinning slightly, and she was gaining weight, even though her appetite was actually decreasing. Bette also began to feel depressed and found it difficult to concentrate. At first she thought that these symptoms might be caused by menopause, but when her neck began to swell noticeably she went to see her doctor.

The doctor found that her skin was extremely pale, cold, dry, and scaly, especially on her elbows and knees. Her pulse was slow and her tendon reflexes were slow to relax. Her thyroid gland was definitely enlarged. A blood sample revealed low thyroid hormone levels and confirmed the doctor's suspicions that Bette was suffering from hypothyroidism. He prescribed thyroid replacement therapy, starting with 25 micrograms daily of thyroxine, and building up to 0.15 milligrams daily over a period of three months. Six months after this diagnosis and treatment, Bette was free of her symptoms and felt fine again.

SIGNS AND SYMPTOMS
INFANTILE HYPOTHYROIDISM:

Symptoms include: a pot belly, lethargy, dry thickened skin, goiter, difficulty in getting the baby to eat, weak muscles, constipation, a hoarse cry, and an enlarged tongue. Mental retardation and short stature will occur if treatment is delayed.

JUVENILE HYPOTHYROIDISM:
Symptoms are: short stature, mental slowness (which is reversible with treatment), dry skin and hair, sometimes excessive growth of hair on the face and body, and often goiter and anemia.

ADULT HYPOTHYROIDISM:
The onset of this disorder is slow and insidious and may not be recognized until a year or more after it begins. Symptoms may include any of the following:

- Cold intolerance (preferring warm rooms, exhibiting a tendency to overdress, and sleeping with blankets even during the summer months);
- Puffy face (especially around the eyes);
- Hoarseness of the voice;
- Deafness;
- Sensations of numbness and tingling in the hands and feet;
- Puffiness of the backs of the hands and tops of the feet;
- Pain in the wrist, and weakness and soreness of the thumb muscle;
- Weight gain despite a normal appetite and diet;
- Heavy periods that may cause anemia;
- High blood cholesterol, leading to hardening of the arteries and angina;
- Flushed cheeks;
- Yellow-tinged skin;
- Dry, cold, rough, and hairless skin;
- Generalized aches and pains;
- Thickened lips;
- Wire-like hair, and/or loss of hair;
- Slow pulse;
- High blood pressure;
- Psychosis in severe cases, but more commonly some apathy, poor memory, and slowness of thought and reactions; and
- if subjected to stress (particularly cold environmental temperatures) or central nervous system depressants such as sedatives, the untreated hypothyroid patient can go into a coma.

METHODS OF DIAGNOSIS

The physician can usually diagnose hypothyroidism based on the signs and symptoms mentioned above, but she confirms the diagnosis by taking a blood sample and measuring the levels of thyroid hormones, as well as TSH levels and the levels of antibodies to thyroid tissue. There are two forms of thyroid hormone: T3 (triiodothyronine) is the active hormone and T4 (thyroxine) is the inactive one. Though both are produced by the thyroid gland from iodine and passed out into the bloodstream, other tissues, especially those of the liver, can convert T4 to T3. Patients with hypothyroidism show low T4 levels and raised TSH levels. Since the latter is the earliest indicator of the disease, some patients may have normal T4 readings but raised TSH readings, which means that the disease has just started to develop. T3 readings are not good indicators, since they may be low for other reasons, such as when the body is unable to convert T4 to T3 due to illness, major surgery, or drug use. If the patient has a high level of antibodies to thyroid tissue in the blood, then he is diagnosed as having Hashimoto's disease.

TREATMENT

Treatment of hypothyroidism requires lifelong thyroxine therapy. Patients are usually started on 25 or 50 micrograms daily and gradually increased at three- to four-week intervals over a three-month period to 100 to 200 micrograms daily. The final adjustment of the thyroxine dosage is made by measuring T3, T4, and TSH levels after the patient has been on the medication for those three months. If the T4 and TSH levels are normal, then the dosage is correct. However, if the T3 and T4 levels are abnormally high, and the TSH levels are low, then the person is overmedicated and the dosage is reduced. Once the correct dosage is found, it may be left constant for years, with the doctor checking blood levels once a year to make sure they remain normal.

IMPOTENCE

DEFINITION

Impotence is defined as a man's inability to develop or sustain an erection long enough to enable him to have sexual intercourse and ejaculation. This condition may be persistent and caused by an imbalance or illness (in which case the man never sustains an erection); or it can be intermittent, where the man cannot always get an erection when he desires it, as in the case of the nervous jitters often called "honeymoon impotence."

HOW COMMON IS IT?

One-third of all middle-aged men suffer from some form of impotence, and the incidence increases with age: 50 percent of all seventy-year-olds have the problem.

CAUSES

The most common causes of impotence are a lack of libido (the physiological and mental drive to attain sexual satisfaction) or short-term physical illnesses like pneumonia, hepatitis, and so forth. In most of the former cases the problem is psychological, proved by the fact that these men can usually still get erections in the early morning. Emotional problems of this nature can be caused by a prior history of embarrassing social or sexual experiences, dissatisfaction with one's work or accomplishments, an unsatisfying home life, fatigue from overwork, lack of communication with one's sexual partner, depression, or other psychiatric disorders. Impotence can also be due to a physical illness, or the use of certain medications including cimetidine, spironolactone, beta blockers, methyldopa, estrogens, phenothiazines, thiazides, tricyclic antidepressants, digoxin, reserpine, and alcohol.

More serious physical causes of impotence are often due to disorders of the blood supply to the penis. (The blood supply is responsible for the erection.) These disorders include diabetes, poor circulation through the arteries in the lower part of the body, multiple sclerosis and spinal cord tumors. Other possible causes are: immature or poorly-functioning testes; high levels of prolactin; surgery in the area of the testes (removal of the prostate); damage or disease of the penis; a serious infection in the urethra (the tube connecting the bladder to the penis); or an overactive thyroid.

CASE HISTORY

Matthew had been a diabetic since his college days but he refused to let the disease ruin his life. He was married and had two healthy, fine looking children. But now, at age 50, he was finding it very difficult to get an erection, even though he was still extremely interested in sex. His wife first tried to ignore it for his sake, but as she saw her husband becoming more and depressed about the problem, she began to urge him to see a doctor. Matthew felt somewhat embarrassed and put it off, though he continued worrying about it.

When it was time for his next checkup, he casually mentioned to his doctor that he was having some problem in this area. The doctor sat Matthew down and explained that unfortunately the diabetes was responsible. "Diabetes causes arteriosclerosis or hardening of the arteries," the doctor said. "When this happens in the arteries supplying the penis an insufficient amount of blood flows into the organ when the man becomes aroused, making it impossible for him to obtain and then maintain an erection."

The doctor told Matthew that the problem would probably become worse until he would eventually be unable to get an erection at all. Unfortunately, there was nothing the doctor could do for him. He didn't tell Matthew that he was one of the more unfortunate diabetics, since most are able to have normal sexual relations throughout their lives.

SIGNS AND SYMPTOMS

The inability to get an erection and maintain it through sexual intercourse. In some situations, a man finds himself able to get an erection but not to ejaculate. This is most often due to fatigue or alcoholism.

METHODS OF DIAGNOSIS

The reason for the patient's impotence is often easily seen by the doctor after he does a physical examination and takes a medical history. If no obvious cause is found, a blood sample is taken to test levels of testosterone, prolactin, and sometimes LH, although these are rarely found to be abnormal. If thyroid disease is suspected, these levels are tested as well.

TREATMENT

For men with psychologically triggered impotence, professional counseling usually helps solve the problem. In the case of immature testes or low levels of sex hormones, testosterone is given. Patients with abnormally high prolactin levels can be treated with a dopamine-like drug such as bromocriptine. An overactive thyroid is treated with antithyroid drugs or radioactive iodine.

INFERTILITY

DEFINITION

A person qualifies as infertile, or unable to have children, if they have had one to two years of unprotected intercourse (intercourse without the use of any birth control method) without becoming pregnant.

HOW COMMON IS IT?

About 10 to 15 percent of all married couples are unable to have children. The male is responsible for 40 percent of all cases and the female for the other 60 percent. Problems with the fallopian tubes account for 20 to 30 percent; problems with the ovaries, another 10 to 15 percent; abnormal cervical mucus, 5 percent; and the remaining 10 to 20 percent are a mystery. Approximately 15 percent of all couples who cannot have children remain permanently infertile despite medical treatment.

CAUSES

The causes of infertility are so numerous it would be impossible to list all of them here, but the following includes most of the main culprits:

IN THE MALE:
- Raised temperature of the testes due to a varicocele (an enlarged blood vessel supplying the genital area);
- Blockage of the vas deferens or epididymis (tubes in the testes carrying the sperm that eventually ends up in the penis);
- An infection of the genital area such as gonorrhea, tuberculosis, urethritis (an infection in the urethra), or mumps;
- Toxins such as cannabis (marijuana), alcohol, opiates;
- Use of drugs such as chemotherapeutic medications, cimetidine, nitrofurantoin, spironolactone, sulfasalazine, androgens;
- Environmental toxins such as pesticides, insecticides, lead, cadmium;
- Radiation therapy;
- Genetic defects in the structure of the genitals or in their development which cause inadequate levels of gonadotropins, such as in Klinefelter's syndrome;

- Antisperm antibodies present in the body;
- Hypothalamic and/or pituitary disorders;
- Thyroid disease (discussed in the Guide) or other chronic diseases;
- Impotence (the preceding section of the Guide);
- Premature ejaculation.

IN THE FEMALE:
- Blockages in the fallopian tubes;
- An unruptured hymen;
- An infection of the genital area such as gonorrhea, or pelvic inflammatory disease;
- Endometriosis;
- Polycystic ovarian disease (discussed in Hirsutism section of the Guide);
- Premature menopause;
- Ovarian tumors;
- Hypothalamic and/or pituitary disorders;
- Use of drugs such as phenothiazines, met clopramide, haloperidol, pimozide, reserpine, methyldopa;
- Thyroid disease (Hypo- and Hyperthyroidism and Thyroid Nodules, discussed in the Guide);
- Adrenal disease (see Adrenocorticol Insufficiency, Cushing's Syndrome, Pheochromocytoma, and Primary Aldosteronism);
- Amenorrhea (discussed in the Guide);
- Antisperm antibodies in the cervical mucus.

CASE HISTORY

Marjorie James started taking oral contraceptives when she was eighteen years old but stopped using them when she turned twenty-two because she broke up with her childhood sweetheart. However, she went to a party shortly afterwards and made love to a stranger there without using any birth control because she felt so alone and confused. To her dismay, she became pregnant. Ten weeks later she had an abortion, which was followed by heavy bleeding and a fever beginning six days afterwards. She returned to the hospital, where they removed the remains of the products of conception and treated her with antibiotics.

In order to prevent another unwanted pregnancy, she had herself fitted with an intrauterine device (IUD). However, it caused her to have heavy periods and after a year she developed stomach pains. The IUD was removed. She then went back on the pill until she was married at the age of twenty-eight, when she stopped taking it in the hopes of becoming pregnant. Although her periods were normal for the next three years she failed to conceive a child.

Her husband was tested for infertility but was found to be fine. Marjorie then went to her doctor, who told her to keep a temperature chart. The chart showed a one degree rise in the second half of her cycle, proving that she was ovulating normally. A test done on her cervical mucus also indicated that there were a normal number of active sperm present in her cervical canal.

The doctor now suspected that Marjorie's fallopian tubes were blocked, probably as a result of the infection she suffered after her abortion and the IUD. This diagnosis was confirmed by a procedure called laparoscopy and hydrotubation, where a blue dye is injected into the uterus, and the fallopian tubes are observed for the appearance of the dye at the ovarian end. The dye did not appear in Marjorie's case, suggesting that her tubes were indeed blocked. This was further confirmed by another procedure called a hysterosalpingography, which is an X-ray examination where a radioactive dye is used in place of the blue dye.

The blockages in Marjorie's fallopian tubes were found to be relatively minor and were freed by surgery. One year after that surgery, Marjorie became pregnant. She and her husband now have three children.

SIGNS AND SYMPTOMS

The inability to have children even though no method of birth control is used.

METHODS OF DIAGNOSIS

IN THE MALE:

The man is told to masturbate into a warm glass container after three days of not having sex. The semen is then analyzed within one hour of its collection. This is repeated at the same time each month for three consecutive months. If the man has an illness which causes raised body temperature, these tests are delayed until he recovers, since raised temperatures (whether from an illness, a hot bath, or an enlarged vein) impair the production of sperm. After the temperature has returned to normal, it takes seventy-four days for sperm to be produced and reach full maturity.

If the sperm are found to be normal and the count of sperm normal after these tests are done, further investigation is usually done on the female partner.

If the sperm do not move very well, the doctor will then check for the presence of antisperm antibodies. If the sperm count is low, prolactin and FSH levels are measured. A high prolactin or low FSH level indicates a problem with the hypothalamus or pituitary. A high prolactin level alone can be caused by thyroid disease, although in these cases other symptoms of the disease will be present to aid in diagnosis (see Thyroid sections of the Guide). A high FSH level alone could mean that the testes are abnormal. Normal FSH levels might suggest the presence of a varicocele, which can be confirmed by measuring the blood supply throughout the testes. A normal FSH level could also indicate a blockage in the vas deferens, which can then be further investigated.

IN THE FEMALE:

A basal body temperature chart is kept to see if the woman is ovulating properly. The temperature is taken upon awakening in the morning and the woman writes down when she menstruates. A woman normally ovulates on the fourteenth day of her cycle and this is followed by a rise in body temperature which is maintained until menstruation fourteen days later. If the temperature does not rise during the proper time by at least one-half degree Celsius then the woman is probably not ovulating. This can be confirmed by taking a blood sample to analyze progesterone levels between the twenty-first and twenty-third days of the cycle. An adequate rise in these levels indicates that ovulation has taken place. If the rise is not adequate, LH, FSH, and prolactin levels are measured, along with thyroid levels if there is any other symptom of thyroid disease (see Thyroid sections of the Guide).

A high reading of FSH and LH could indicate premature menopause or a problem with the ovaries. A low FSH and LH level, or a high prolactin level could suggest a problem with the pituitary or hypothalamus. High prolactin levels can also mean thyroid disease. A lack of ovulation when there are normal LH and FSH levels present might mean a lack of progesterone.

If a woman ovulates normally she is then tested to make sure her fallopian tubes are not blocked. In addition, a test is done on her cervical mucus within twelve to sixteen hours after sexual intercourse in order to make sure there is an adequate amount of live sperm remaining in the cervical canal. A normal test result rules out any cervical factor. An abnormal test is usually repeated within one to three hours after intercourse.

TREATMENT
IN THE MALE:

Men with low sperm counts should avoid taking hot baths and wearing tightly fitting underwear and trousers. All factors causing excess prolactin production are corrected (such as tumors of the pituitary, the use of certain medications, hyperthyroidism). Antibiotics are given to cure infections of the genitals. Gonadotropin deficiency is treated with GnRH or HCG. Blockages in the vas deferens can be removed although this is often not successful. The presence of sperm antibodies can be treated with the drug prednisone.

IN THE FEMALE:

An unruptured hymen can be surgically removed. Infections in the reproductive organs can be treated with the appropriate antibiotics. Fallopian tube blockages can be surgically removed but this is not always successful. Patients producing too little progesterone to thicken the walls of the uterus for implantation of the ovum (egg) may increase their production of the hormone when injected with bromocriptine or HCG. Women with elevated prolactin levels can usually be treated with bromocriptine. Tumors producing excess prolactin may be removed surgically or treated with radiotherapy.

Women with high prolactin levels due to thyroid disease can be cured by correcting the thyroid problem. Women who are not ovulating are treated with clomiphene and if that is not successful, gonadotropins are administered. If a woman had antibodies to sperm in her cervical mucus, the use of a condom during intercourse for six months will reduce the antibody level and successful fertilization may occur when the condom is not used. Corticosteroid therapy or artificial insemination by the husband are alternative treatments for the woman if the condom method is not effective.

OSTEOPOROSIS

DEFINITION

People with osteoporosis lose abnormal amounts of bone as they get older, making the bones brittle and prone to fractures.

HOW COMMON IS IT?

Fifteen to twenty million Americans, or one in every three to four middle-aged or older people have osteoporosis. It can occur in anyone over the age of forty-five but is particularly prevalent among postmenopausal women of British, Northern European, Chinese, Japanese, or Jewish extraction. Black women are in a low-risk group for the disease.

CAUSES

Bones are continuously being broken down and reformed. Up until about the age of forty, bone formation proceeds at a faster rate than bone breakdown and so the bone continuously increases in strength and density. After age forty, people lose more bone than they make, and so the bones become more brittle and porous. The rate of bone loss is more rapid in women than in men, especially after menopause. In people who develop osteoporosis, this process proceeds at a faster rate than normal.

The risk for getting the disease is affected by a number of factors concerned with bone formation and breakdown. The things that increase bone formation in early life will decrease the chance of getting the disease and the things that increase bone loss will increase the risk for osteoporosis.

Inadequate amounts of calcium and vitamin D in the diet for the first four decades of life will reduce the amount of bone made in the body during these years. This will mean that less bone has to be lost before a person is said to have osteoporosis. Some elderly people cannot convert vitamin D to its active form and so are unable to absorb calcium from their meals, which leads to rapid bone loss and osteoporosis.

If a person has been confined to bed for a long time, has spent a lot of time in a wheelchair, or leads a very sedentary life, she is at greater risk for getting the disease. This is because activities like walking, running, or standing cause the muscles to pull on the skeleton which is a stimulus to bone formation.

Estrogen also stimulates bone formation, which means that a woman who goes into menopause early can have a greater risk for developing osteoporosis. Obese postmenopausal women have greater protection because fat tissue converts androgens into estrogens. To a lesser extent, reduced levels of male sex hormones in a man also leads to bone loss.

Other causes of accelerated bone loss include excessive alcohol consumption, cigarette smoking, an overactive thyroid, Cushing's syndrome, diabetes mellitus (both discussed in the Guide) and treatment with large doses of corticosteroids.

CASE HISTORY
Anne Forsythe was a sixty-year-old owner of a small but successful publishing company. Throughout her life she had invested all her energies in the business that she had inherited from her father. Having a small and frail frame, she had always despised any form of physical activity.

Anne developed ovarian cancer when she was forty-one and was given a hysterectomy. Over the last few years, she had suffered from chronic backaches and had noticed that her posture wasn't as straight as it used to be. She did not consult a doctor, since she believed her problems were caused by the long hours she spent hunched over her desk, reading and editing manuscripts.

One winter she slipped on the ice and broke her wrist. The X-ray taken at the hospital showed that Anne was suffering from osteoporosis. Her doctor gave her a calcium supplement and put her on hormone replacement therapy, using a mixture of estrogen and progesterone. He also encouraged her to walk as much as possible instead of driving everywhere and to climb stairs rather than take the elevator, as well as to stop smoking and drinking. One year later, using a technique called photon absorptiometry, the doctor found that Anne's bones had gotten a little stronger.

SIGNS AND SYMPTOMS
Bones become very brittle, especially in the spinal cord, hip, thigh bone, and wrist, and so tend to fracture more easily than normal. As the bones in the spinal cord compress (become crushed), the person has back pain, loss of height, and eventually may end up with a "widow's hump."

METHODS OF DIAGNOSIS
Osteoporosis is not usually diagnosed until a person has had it for a

significant amount of time. X-rays are not sensitive enough to detect a decrease of bone until there is enough loss to cause a clinical problem such as back pain or a fracture. By that time X-rays show decreased bone density in the skull, spine, and long bones (especially in the bones of the hand). A bone biopsy will confirm the loss.

TREATMENT

In males, androgens, and in females, estrogens, can be given to retard the progression of the disease; however, women must take the estrogen with progesterone to prevent the development of endometrial cancer. This treatment may restart menstrual bleeding in elderly women, which many find unacceptable. Adequate amounts of vitamin D should be consumed through the diet, and elderly people may be given supplements of active vitamin D if they cannot produce it themselves. A calcium intake of 1500 milligrams a day is strongly recommended. Weight-bearing exercise such as walking, jogging, cycling, and tennis may prevent the condition from getting worse. By following these strategies, pain may improve and further loss in height prevented. Analgesics can be taken for the pain.

The progression of the disease is monitored by using a technique called photon absorptiometry, which can measure very small changes in bone density.

PHEOCHROMOCYTOMA

DEFINITION

This disorder is characterized by the oversecretion of epinephrine and/or norepinephrine by the adrenal medulla (which forms the core of the adrenal gland).

HOW COMMON IS IT?

Less than 1 person per 10,000 in the general population have the disease; 1 to 5 people per 1,000 who are under the age of fifty and suffer from high blood pressure have it. In 10 to 20 percent of all cases it runs in families.

CAUSES

In over 80 percent of the cases, this disorder is caused by a tumor in the adrenal medulla that is usually benign. In the remaining people, it is caused by tumors in other areas of the nervous system. About 10 percent of all these tumors are malignant. Sometimes tumors develop in both adrenal glands, especially in children.

CASE HISTORY

Michael Massey was a forty-two-year-old engineer who owned a cement manufacturing plant. He went to see his doctor, complaining of frequent headaches. He explained that they would attack him at any time of the day, caused throbbing pains in the top and front of his head, and lasting for between five minutes and one hour. When the headaches first appeared, they only occurred once every three or four weeks, but during the last month this had increased to once every four or five days. When the headaches came, Michael would begin to sweat, feel nauseous, and his heart would start racing.

The doctor found that Michael had moderately high blood pressure, which, with the other symptoms, made him suspect pheochromocytoma. A urine test revealed high levels of the breakdown products of norepinephrine and epinephrine and so the doctor diagnosed Michael as having a norepinephrine- and epinephrine-producing tumor. A CAT scan showed a single tumor in his right adrenal gland. Michael was given a drug called phenoxybenzamine to block the action of the norepinephrine produced by the tumor and over the next few days his blood pressure gradually returned to normal. The heart symptoms were treated with a drug called propranolol. Surgery was then performed to remove the tumor. Michael's operation was successful and he made a complete recovery.

SIGNS AND SYMPTOMS

The patient has sporadic attacks, lasting for less than one hour, of intense anxiety, palpitations, and finally a throbbing headache. They are usually very pale and sweat heavily during these attacks, which leave them completely exhausted. Nausea, vomiting, and stomach pains may also accompany the attacks. These unpleasant episodes may be provoked by physical exertion, emotional stresses, or by bending or twisting the body.

Symptoms such as high blood pressure, sweating, and headaches are due to the oversecretion of norepinephrine; heart symptoms such as palpitations are caused by epinephrine excess.

METHODS OF DIAGNOSIS

The majority of people with pheochromocytoma have high blood pressure at all times, which increases to even higher levels during the attacks described above. About 25 percent have high blood pressure only during these attacks. The combination of high blood pressure with spells of sweating, headache, and palpitations often means that the person has a norepinephrine- and/or epinephrine-secreting tumor. Such a diagnosis is confirmed by finding abnormally high levels of the breakdown products of norepinephrine and epinephrine in the urine, and by locating tumors (all types) with a CAT scan or other radiographic procedures.

TREATMENT

Before surgery can be carried out to remove the tumor, the person's blood pressure must be brought down to normal with phenoxybenzamine. This usually takes a few days. Once this has been achieved, palpitations and irregular heart beats are corrected with propranolol or lidocaine. The tumor is then removed. After the surgery, blood pressure may drop below normal since it takes a little time for the body to adjust to the absence of the high doses of norepinephrine produced by the tumor. This is corrected by giving the patient plasma or a saline solution intravenously. People who have malignant tumors that cannot be removed are treated with phenoxybenzamine.

PRECOCIOUS PUBERTY

DEFINITION

Although the onset of puberty can occur as early as age five or six, and there have been reports of girls at age six becoming pregnant, sexual maturation in a boy under the age of nine or in a girl under the age of eight must be called precocious and is caused by the premature release of GnRH, sometimes due to an underlying physical disorder.

When a child suffers from precocious puberty, he or she may either develop the appropriate characteristics for their sex—a deep voice, heavier muscular structure, and enlargement of the penis for a boy; breasts and menstrual periods for a girl—or the child may develop inappropriate characteristics, as in the masculine traits appearing in women with adrenal gland tumors.

Precocity is further divided into true precocity, where a boy or girl develops sexual characteristics along with the full maturation of the ovaries or testes, or false precocity, where the sexual characteristics appear but the ovaries or testes do not mature at the same rate.

HOW COMMON IS IT?

One in 5000 children have some form of precocious sexual maturation. It is five times more common in girls than in boys. In 10 percent of all cases it runs in families (a woman who sexually matures at eleven might find her daughter maturing at age eight). In 80 percent of the cases in girls and 50 percent in boys, this early puberty develops in a normal manner, only at a younger age than usual. The remaining 20 percent of girls and 50 percent of boys are suffering from an underlying disorder.

CAUSES

True precosity: Children who develop early but normally do so because of the premature release of GnRH from the hypothalamus. Those who have an underlying disorder may be suffering from an infection in the hypothalamic area of the brain (such as encephalitis or meningitis), a tumor in the pineal gland or hypothalamus, hypothyroidism affecting the hypothalamus, or tumors in other parts of the body that produce gonadotropins.

False precocity: This condition always indicates a disorder and can be caused by congenital (existing at birth) defects in the adrenal glands, an adrenal gland tumor, Cushing's syndrome (resulting from the excess production of cortisol), or tumors in the ovaries or testes.

CASE HISTORY

Samantha June was a perfect baby. She weighed over seven pounds at birth and seemed perfectly healthy in every way. She was a happy child, a delight to her parents, and rarely ever sick. But at the age of five, her mother was bathing her and noticed small hairs developing on her pubic region and under her arms. Around this same time, Samantha started growing at an alarmingly fast rate. At first her parents were worried but not frantic, but then Samantha began to develop the first signs of breasts. One day her mother found her in the bathroom sobbing. "Mommy, I'm bleeding," the small child cried. Her mother looked and saw that her baby girl was menstruating. She took Samantha Jane to her pediatrician the very next day.

The doctor did a CAT scan (a scan of the brain) and measured the child's hormonal levels. Since all these tests proved normal, he diagnosed Samantha as having true precocity with no underlying disorder. She was treated with a drug called medroxy progesterone acetate. Her breasts did get smaller, she stopped menstruating, but she still continued to grow at a faster rate than normal for her age. Today, Samantha June is a healthy woman who stands well under five feet.

SIGNS AND SYMPTOMS

In Girls: Breast enlargement, hair in the armpits, growth of pubic hair, menstrual bleeding. The bones grow rapidly and then stop growing prematurely, leaving the girl with a short stature. If androgens are involved, they develop deepening of the voice and enlargement of the clitoris.

In Boys: Early growth of pubic and underarm hair, enlargement of the penis, development of extra muscle, and deepening of the voice. Their skeletons grow rapidly and then stop growing prematurely, stunting their growth. When estrogen excess is involved, they develop breasts.

METHODS OF DIAGNOSIS

True precocity: Doctors examine the brain with X-rays or other techniques producing images of the brain such as nuclear magnetic resonance (NMR) or a CAT scan. These will show up any evidence of a tumor. Thyroxine and TSH levels in the blood should be measured to rule out hypothyroidism, and blood gonadotropin levels tested to rule out gonadotropin-producing tumors.

False precocity: Urinary and blood plasma analysis for steroids produced by the adrenals is done to rule out congenital adrenal problems. Plasma and urine cortisol levels are tested to eliminate Cushing's syndrome. Plasma testosterone is checked to see if there are tumors of the testes and "masculinizing" tumors of the ovaries.

TREATMENT

True precocity: Rapid sexual development may be retarded by giving the child antigonadotropin drugs such as medroxy progesterone acetate, cyproterone acetate (not yet available in the U.S.), or GnRH analogs. (Analogs are substances similar in nature and action to the original compound but with a slightly different structure.) These drugs inhibit the secretion of GnRH or the pituitary's response to GnRH. They decrease menstruation and breast size, but the bones continue to grow at an accelerated rate and then stop growing prematurely, causing short stature. Reassurance and psychological treatment are also needed, as premature sexual development can be very upsetting to the child.

False precocity: Treatment involves correcting the underlying physical defect, such as surgically removing any tumors, giving cortisol to children with congenitally enlarged adrenal glands, or giving thyroxine when hypothyroidism exists.

PRIMARY ALDOSTERONISM (CONN'S SYNDROME)

DEFINITION
This disorder involves a higher than normal secretion of the adrenocortical hormone aldosterone, which helps maintain blood pressure and normal concentrations of sodium in the body.

HOW COMMON IS IT?
Less than 1 in 10,000 people in the general population have it, but between 1 and 5 per 1,000 of those under the age of 50 with high blood pressure suffer from the disease. It occasionally runs in families.

CAUSES
In 80 percent of all cases, Conn's syndrome is due to an aldosterone-producing tumor (adenoma) in the adrenal cortex. Such tumors are much more common in women than in men.

In the other cases, it is caused by a spontaneous growth of cells that produce aldosterone in the adrenal cortex of both adrenal glands (called bilateral adrenal hyperplasia).

CASE HISTORY
Peter Brown, thirty-five, a high school French teacher, went to his doctor complaining of general weakness, which he estimated had gotten gradually worse over the last two and a half years. He was now suffering from muscle cramps as well, which had recently started. During the last eighteen months he was having to get up at night to urinate but was not any more thirsty than normal.

The doctor found that Peter's blood pressure was higher than it should be. His blood tests showed low potassium and renin levels. This made the doctor suspect Conn's syndrome, and Peter was admitted to the hospital for more tests. He was given a saline solution (which contains sodium) intravenously and his urine was collected over a twenty-four-hour period. The urine showed an abnormally high aldosterone content and so the diagnosis was confirmed. A CAT scan revealed that Peter had a benign tumor on his left adrenal gland. He was given potassium supplements and spironolactone (a diuretic that counteracts the effects of aldosterone) for a two-week period in order to build up his potassium stores. He was then operated on and the tumor was removed. Peter is now completely cured.

SIGNS AND SYMPTOMS

Periods of extreme muscle weakness, muscle cramps, lethargy, frequent urination, and higher than normal blood pressure causing headaches and shortness of breath.

METHODS OF DIAGNOSIS

A blood workup is done on people with high blood pressure, and if low blood potassium levels are found and the person is not taking diuretics (diuretics deplete the body of potassium), then Conn's syndrome is suspected.

Blood renin levels are also low. When the blood pressure goes down in a normal person, the kidneys produce renin which is indirectly responsible for stimulating the adrenal glands to produce aldosterone, which raises blood pressure. In a person with Conn's syndrome, aldosterone production is high regardless of the levels of renin.

The diagnosis is confirmed by measuring the amount of aldosterone in the urine passed over a twenty-four hour period by a person given sodium intravenously. Sodium given to a normal person in this way would decrease the amount of aldosterone made by the adrenals, which, in turn, would reduce the amount of aldosterone found in the urine. However, in the Conn's syndrome patient, the aldosterone in the urine remains abnormally high despite the presence of high levels of sodium in the body.

Once the doctor has established that the person had Conn's syndrome, he then must find the cause. This can be done by using a CAT scan to seek out the adenoma. But because these tumors can be very small, the scan may not find them. The other possible cause of the disease is overgrown adrenal glands. If a person has this problem, her aldosterone levels will rise when she stands up after lying down for a long time. Therefore, blood levels are measured upon rising in the morning and then four hours later, after the person spends the morning walking around. If the levels rise, overgrown adrenals are causing the problem. If the levels do not rise, then it must be assumed that a very small tumor is the cause. By taking samples of the blood coming from each adrenal gland, the doctor can determine which one is producing excess aldosterone and therefore has the tumor.

TREATMENT

People with an adrenal adenoma are given potassium supplements and spironolactone, which has the opposite effect to aldosterone and makes the body excrete sodium and retain potassium. The process takes two to three weeks. The adenoma is then surgically removed. (Potassium stores have to be built back up before surgery, since a person must be in the best condition possible before undergoing an operation, and potassium is needed by the body for proper muscle, nerve, and heart function.)

People with overgrown adrenal glands are treated with spironolactone, which also has the effect of slightly reducing the ability of the adrenal glands to make aldosterone. Spironolactone is also used to treat the elderly and other people who have adrenal adenomas but are not fit (too weak or otherwise ill) for surgery.

RICKETS AND OSTEOMALACIA

DEFINITION

Osteomalacia and rickets are really the same disorder except that osteomalacia affects adults and rickets affects children. The condition is marked by an inability to absorb calcium from the diet. This means that there is less calcium available for deposition into the bones to harden them. Calcium is crucial to most essential body functions, such as the activity of the nervous system and the contraction of the muscles.

HOW COMMON IS IT?

Although this disease appears infrequently in the United States, in some populations as many as one out of ten people have the problem because of a poor diet.

CAUSES

Vitamin D is a hormone made in the skin when a person is exposed to a normal amount of sunlight. The hormone is also found in certain foods, such as fatty fish (herring, salmon, mackerel) and to a lesser extent in eggs, milk, cheese, and butter. Lack of exposure to sunlight as in house bound people or those living in northern latitudes combined with a low intake of foods rich in vitamin D, can lead to this disease.

People with any kind of malabsorption problem causing them to have chronic diarrhea may not be able to absorb enough vitamin D from their food to satisfy the body's needs.

Once vitamin D is absorbed into the body it must be made potent in the liver and then the kidney before it can do its job of facilitating calcium absorption. People with either liver or kidney disease may not be able to carry out these crucial activation steps.

Drugs taken by people with epilepsy (such as diphenylhydantoin and phenobarbitone) speed up the rate at which the body breaks down vitamin D and reduces the liver's activation of the vitamin.

Some people are born with genetic defects that prevent the kidneys from activating vitamin D. The problem usually appears at one year of age when the child begins to walk and causes rickets. Another genetic defect causes children to lose calcium from their bones at a very rapid rate.

People with hyperparathyroidism or hyperthyroidism (both discussed in the Guide) sometimes develop osteomalacia.

CASE HISTORY

Frank DiMellio, a seventy-year-old retired grandfather, frequently took laxatives and so invariably had loose bowel movements. Being a widower, he often missed meals and when he did eat, he preferred cakes and cookies to more nourishing food. Frank also rarely left his house, even in the warmer summer season. During the last month he noticed that he was having difficulty getting in and out of chairs, and when he climbed the stairs he found he had to pull himself up by the bannisters. Frank assumed at first that his symptoms were just another part of aging, but his friends finally convinced him to see a doctor.

The doctor gave him a thorough physical examination and found some degree of muscle weakness. A blood test revealed that Frank had low calcium levels and high alkaline phosphatase levels. Since the doctor suspected osteomalacia, he sent Frank to the hospital for a series of x-rays. These showed lines of uncalcified bone tissue across his hip bones and at the top of his thigh bones, which confirmed the diagnosis.

The doctor weaned Frank off laxatives by getting him to eat a bowl of bran cereal every morning for breakfast. He also gave him vitamin D and calcium supplements. Within one month Frank was feeling much stronger and more able to get around.

SIGNS AND SYMPTOMS

Rickets: Children with this disorder have very soft bones. Because of their low calcium absorption they may be irritable and may even have tetany (where the muscles are severely contracted and immobile) or convulsions. The soft bones leads to bowing of the arms in crawling babies and of the legs in children. Children may also waddle when they walk. A number of lumps may be felt where the ribs join the sternum; the growth of the child's skeleton and teeth will be delayed; and the children will be stunted in height.

Osteomalacia: The adult will have pains and aches in the bones that tend to start in the pelvic area and spread to the spine and ribs. If the disease is not treated the person will begin to stoop and will break bones more easily than normal. They may also suffer from muscular weakness.

METHODS OF DIAGNOSIS

In people with this disease, blood calcium levels are usually subnormal or in the lower half of the normal range. Blood phosphate levels are also low. An enzyme called alkaline phosphatase is usually elevated in the blood: this enzyme breaks down bone to liberate calcium into the blood and so in times of dietary shortage or impaired absorption the mineral is obtained from the bones via the actions of this enzyme.

Blood levels of vitamin D are low both in people who are deficient in the vitamin and those with liver or kidney problems. The X-rays of a patient with osteomalacia will show strips of uncalcified bone tissue in the ribs, across the pelvis, at the pelvic ends of the thigh bones, and along the edge of the shoulder blades. In the case of rickets, the growing ends of the bones are enlarged. Bone biopsies (where a piece of bone is surgically removed) may be needed if the diagnosis is in doubt; in people with the disease these will show abnormally low quantities of calcium deposited into the tissue.

TREATMENT
Supplements of calcium and vitamin D (or activated vitamin D) are given, and the symptoms gradually disappear.

THYROID NODULES
(INCLUDING THYROID CANCER)

DEFINITION
Thyroid nodules are lumps in the thyroid gland which can be:
- Associated with hyperthyroidism;
- Fluid-filled sacs called cysts; or
- Cancerous growths.

When there are only one or two lumps present in the gland, there is a much greater chance that they may be cancerous.

HOW COMMON IS IT?
Thyroid nodules are five times more common in women than in men (5 per 100 as opposed to 1 per 100), but a man with a thyroid nodule is more likely to have thyroid cancer. In children, thyroid nodules are extremely rare but about half of them are cancerous.

The risk of getting thyroid cancer, which tends to run in families, is extremely small. There are only thirty-nine new cases per one million people each year.

CAUSES
The causes of thyroid nodules are for the most part unknown. However, thyroid cancer does seem to occur more frequently in people whose head and neck have been exposed to a large number of X-rays. After exposure to the radiation, it takes an average of twenty years before the cancer develops, but it can take anywhere from five to thirty-five years.

CASE HISTORY
Jim Green, a forty-one-year-old business executive, went for a physical demanded by his new place of employment. There the doctors found a small lump in his neck, and he was told that he could not be approved for the firm's insurance policy until he was checked out by an endocrinologist. Jim went to see a thyroid specialist who again examined his neck and found a hard lump within the thyroid gland. He

scheduled Jim for a scintiscan and found the lump to be "cold." The doctor now suspected cancer. Blood tests revealed that Jim's thyroid gland was producing normal amounts of hormones. When Jim told the doctor that he had been given extensive X-rays when he was a child for recurrent tonsillitis, the doctor explained that this could have caused cancer. This suspicion was confirmed when the doctor performed a biopsy on Jim's thyroid.

Jim was sent to a surgeon specializing in the thyroid who removed the gland. One month after surgery he was given radioactive iodine to destroy any remaining thyroid tissue that could potentially grow into another lump. He was then given thyroid hormone and checked six months later to make sure there was no remaining thyroid tissue and no evidence of the cancer having spread to other parts of his body. Fortunately, he was fine. Eighteen months after that, Jim was checked again and all was well. Now he goes back to his endocrinologist once a year to have his neck examined and his blood levels of thyroid hormones checked to make sure the dose of thyroxine he takes each day is enough to keep him in the normal range.

SIGNS AND SYMPTOMS

Thyroid cancer is usually marked by a single, painless, rapidly-enlarging lump in the neck which is irregular in shape and fixed in position. (Two enlarging hard lumps in the neck would also be highly suspicious.) It is often associated with hoarseness, a dry cough, difficulty in swallowing, and sometimes problems in catching one's breath.

A generally enlarged gland or one with many lumps is unlikely to be cancerous and more likely to be a sign of Hashimoto's disease (see hypothyroidism in the Guide) or toxic multinodular goiter (see Hyperthyroidism in the Guide).

METHODS OF DIAGNOSIS

A patient who seems to have a single thyroid lump is given a thyroid scintiscan. Here the patient is injected with a small amount of radioactive iodine and an X-ray is taken of the thyroid. The more active the thyroid tissue is in making thyroid hormones, the more iodine it absorbs, since thyroid hormones are made from iodine. Cancerous thyroid tissue does not make thyroid hormone and so does not absorb the iodine. Therefore, when radioactive iodine is injected into the patient, any lump in the thyroid that is cancerous will not absorb the administered iodine and that area of the gland will appear as transparent on the X-ray. It is said to be a "cold" area and the doctor will assume that it may be cancerous. However, if a single lump absorbs a lot of the iodine this means that it is producing a great deal of thyroid hormone and the patient probably has toxic adenoma (see Hyperthyroidism in the Guide). In this case the X-ray will show a very dark area which is said to be "hot."

If the doctor finds a "cold" lump he must make sure that it is cancerous and not a nonmalignant cyst; 20 percent of "cold" lumps do turn out to be cysts. While malignant tumors are solid, cysts are filled with fluid. The doctor can test the lump in two ways. He can do an ultrasound test, which passes sound waves through the thyroid gland. This differentiates between hollow and solid objects. He can also pass a needle into the center of the lump and remove some of the fluid present, and/or some of the cells (a procedure known as a biopsy), which can then be examined for cancer.

When there are many lumps in the thyroid gland, the doctor would examine the patient for signs and symptoms of hyperthyroidism and measure the patient's blood levels of thyroid hormones.

TREATMENT

The best treatment for thyroid cancer is removal of as much of the thyroid tissue as is possible without damaging the laryngeal nerves (involved in speaking) and the parathyroid glands (which lie on top of the thyroid and are involved in controlling the way the body uses calcium). The surgery is followed by treatment with radioactive iodine to destroy any remaining thyroid tissue. The person is then maintained on thyroid hormone replacement therapy, and the thyroid is checked each year to make sure that a problem with the gland does not recur.

Nonmalignant cysts are usually drained. For treatment of nodules associated with hyperthyroidism, (see the Hyperthyroidism section of the Guide).

BIBLIOGRAPHY

Burch, W. M. *Endocrinology for the House Officer* Baltimore: Williams and Williams, 1984.

Edwards, C.R.W. *Integrated Clinical Science: Endocrinology* London: William Heinemann Medical Books Ltd., 1986.

Fletcher, R. F. *Lecture Notes on Endocrinology,* 4th ed. Boston: Blackwell Scientific Publications, 1983.

Gillmer, M., Gordon D., Sever, P., and Steer, P. *One Hundred Cases for Students of Medicine* New York: Churchill Livingstone, 1984.

Gupta, K. L. *Case Studies in Medicine* New York: Churchill Livingstone, 1986.

Hartog, M. *Endocrinology* Boston: Blackwell Scientific Publications, 1987.

Hedge, G. A., Colby H. D., and Goodman, R. L. *Clinical Endocrine Physiology* Philadelphia: W. B. Saunders Co., 1987.

Hershman, J. M. *Endocrine Pathophysiology: A Patient-Oriented Approach,* 3rd. ed. Philadelphia: Lea and Febiger, 1988.

Hind, C.R.R. *Short Cases for the MRCP* New York: Churchill Livingstone, 1984.

Jubiz, W. *Endocrinology: A Logical Approach for Physicians*, 2nd ed. New York: McGraw-Hill Book Co., 1985.

Plowman, P. N. *Endocrinology and Metabolic Diseases* New York: John Wiley and Sons, 1987.

Pounder, R. E. *Long Cases in General Medicine* Boston: Blackwell Scientific Publications, 1983.

Rubenstein, D., Wayne, D. *Lecture Notes on Clinical Medicine*, 3rd ed. Boston: Blackwell Scientific Publications, 1985.

Rumsey, I. *A Synopsis of Endocrinology and Metabolism*, 3rd ed. Bristol: I.O.P. Publishing Ltd., 1986.

Spalton, D. J., Sever P. S., Ward, P. D., Armitstead, J. and Greenstone, M. *One Hundred Case Histories for the MRCP*, 2nd ed. New York: Churchill Livingstone, 1982.

Wise, P. H. *Endocrinology* New York: Churchill Livingstone, 1986.

INDEX

A

Abnormal Growth, *see*
Acromegaly; Gigantism
Accutane, *see* Isotretinoin
Achlorhydria, 30
Acne, 96-97
Acromegaly, 63; *see also*
Gigantism
case history, causes, com-
monality, defined, diagnosis,
signs and symptoms, treat-
ment, 125-27
ACTH, *see* Adrenocorticotro-
pin Hormone
Actin, 20
Addison's Disease, 98
case history, causes, com-
monality, defined, diagnosis,
signs and symptoms, treat-
ment, 128-31
Adenoma (benign tumor)
hyperparathyroidism and,
160, 162
ADH, *see* Vasopressin
Adolescents/Children

adrenal medulla tumor, 187
acne, 96-97
breast development in, 153,
155
Cushing's Syndrome, 137
development and growth,
57-58, 60-61, 125-27, 139,
196
diabetes, 150-51
growth hormones and, 170-71
puberty, 188-89
rickets, 193-96
sex hormones, 68-69
somatomedins, 63
Adolescent Gynecomastia, 153
Adrenal Cortex, 28, 116, 128,
191; *see also* Adrenal
Glands
Adrenal Glands, 20, 26-28,
46, 70, 115-16, 124; *see
also* Aldesterone; Dopamine;
Enkephalins; Epinephrine;
Norepinephrine; Somatostatin;
adenoma, 193
congenitally enlarged, 191

Look for these other fine titles from The Body Press:

Brainfood by Dr. Brian and Roberta Morgan

Diabetic Cooking by Ann Watson and Sue Lousley

The Emotional Pharmacy by Roberta Morgan

Estrogen by Lila Nachtigall, M.D. and Joan Rattner

Food Intolerance by John Hunter, M.D.

HMO's by Jill Bloom

Meganutrients by H.L. Newbold, Ph.D.

Osteoporosis by David Fardon, M.D.

PMS: A Positive Program to Gain Control by Stephanie Bender

PMS: Questions and Answers by Stephanie Bender

Saving Face by Nelson Lee Novick, M.D.

Teenage Body Book by Kathy McCoy and Charles Wibbelsman, M.D.

Young Man's Guide to Sex by Jay Gale, Ph.D

Young Woman's Guide to Sex by Jacqueline Voss, Ph.D and Jay Gale, Ph.D